The Bioanalysis Glossary

In this glossary, 'bioanalysis' is defined as the quantitative or qualitative measurement of endogenous or exogenous analytes in biological matrices. The broader use of the term used by biochemists for biochemical characterization is excluded.

This glossary:

- Lists terms, definitions and equations directly associated with the field of bioanalysis;
- Describes closely related techniques, technologies and applications of bioanalysis, which are important or useful for bioanalysts to understand.
- Covers general bioanalytical terms; (bio)analytical techniques and equipment; pharmacokinetics; clinical trials; metabolomics; antidoping testing; therapeutic drug monitoring; regulatory and validation terminology; drug development; and statistical terminology.

The Bioanalysis Glossary

Edition 2026

Edited by The Glossary Editorial Panel

The Bioanalysis Glossary has been a trusted resource in the field for many years, with its content evolving through six editions in the Taylor & Francis Bioanalysis journal to reflect advancements in bioanalytical science. However, this marks the first time the glossary is being published as a standalone book by CRC Press/Taylor & Francis Group. As such, the publisher is presenting it as the 'First Edition', while acknowledging its rich history and prior iterations. To further distinguish this publication and align it with the current year, we are referring to it as the '2026 Edition'. This designation emphasizes the glossary's relevance and timeliness, ensuring readers understand that it incorporates the latest developments and terminology in bioanalysis.

First edition published 2026
by CRC Press
2385 NW Executive Center Drive, Suite 320, Boca Raton FL 33431

and by CRC Press
4 Park Square, Milton Park, Abingdon, Oxon, OX14 4RN

CRC Press is an imprint of Taylor & Francis Group, LLC

ISBN: 9781041162391 (hbk)
ISBN: 9781041162384 (pbk)
ISBN: 9781003683506 (ebk)

DOI: 10.1201/9781003683506

Typeset in Merriweather
by KnowledgeWorks Global Ltd.

Contents

The Bioanalysis Glossary
6th Edition

November 2025, *Bioanalysis* Vol. 17, No. 23, Suppl. 1

Brought to you by *Bioanalysis* and Bioanalysis Zone

2 Glossary information
3 Sponsors
4 Preface
6 Scope
7 Disclaimer and Copyright Information
8 Terms and definitions
169 Index
179 Company profiles
183 Author guidelines

Publishing information
ISSN 1757-6180

Publication history
First edition published: November 2014
Second edition published: November 2016
Third edition published: November 2018
Fourth edition published: November 2020
Fifth edition published: November 2023
Sixth edition published: November 2025

TAYLOR & FRANCIS

EDITORIAL DEPARTMENT

Bioanalysis

Editor-in-Chief
Neil Spooner
Neil@SpoonerBioanalytical.co.uk

Commissioning Team Manager
Jack Lodge
Jack.Lodge@tandf.co.uk

Bioanalysis Zone

Editor-in-Chief
Naamah Maundrell
Naamah.Maundrell@tandf.co.uk

Senior Editor
Ellen Williams
Ellen.Williams@tandf.co.uk

Editor
Emma Hall
Emma.Hall@tandf.co.uk

Editor
Megan Giboney
Megan.Giboney@tandf.co.uk

Production

New Media Production Supervisor
Kathryn Berry

BUSINESS DEVELOPMENT & SUPPORT

Advertising

Business Development Manager
Lauren Poole
Lauren.Poole@tandf.co.uk

Subscriptions

Business Development Executive
Andrea Fejszes
Andrea.Fejszes@tandf.co.uk

Reprints

Head of Publishing Solutions
Sam Cavana
Sam.Cavana@tandf.co.uk

For *Bioanalysis* submission enquiries, please contact ibio@tandf.co.uk

Sponsors

The Bioanalysis Glossary 6th Edition has been produced in partnership with:

Alturas Analytics
Bioanalytical Experts

celerion
Translating Science to Medicine

Kcas bio
SCIENCE ACCELERATED

WuXi AppTec

2-4 Park Square,
Milton Park,
Abingdon, Oxfordshire,
OX14 4RN, UK

Bioanalysis
the JOURNAL, the ZONE

Taylor & Francis Group
an informa business

Customer Services

Editorial enquiries:
info@bioanalysis-zone.com

Advertising enquiries:
advertising@bioanalysis-zone.com

Preface

The Bioanalysis Glossary

An essential resource for a bioanalyst!

The *Bioanalysis* and Bioanalysis Zone editorial teams are delighted to bring you a new edition of The Bioanalysis Glossary, which continues to be regarded as an essential resource for everyone who works in bioanalysis or adjacent fields. A total of 15 leading experts in the bioanalytical field have been working closely with our editorial teams to provide a comprehensive update to the new edition of our glossary, reflecting the growing field of bioanalysis.

This guide is intended to be of great benefit to individuals who are new to the field or working with bioanalytical laboratories for the first time. Additionally, this glossary serves as a valuable reference for experienced bioanalysts who are working on research papers, reports or presentations. Since its creation, the Bioanalysis Glossary's primary objective has been to facilitate the standardization of terminology used within the bioanalytical community, within and between companies, universities and individuals. In this increasingly globalized field, it has become necessary for scientists to speak the same bioanalytical language.

The glossary encompasses essential bioanalytical terminology to promote consistent usage, along with key terms relevant to various aspects of bioanalysis, such as drug development, metabolomics and therapeutic drug monitoring. This highlights that bioanalysis extends beyond simply generating data. Bioanalysts should actively participate in discussions across all stages of drug development, as a deeper understanding of related fields like pharmacokinetics and the application of data fosters more meaningful and effective bioanalytical practices.

We are very much committed to ensuring we keep moving with this progressive field and stay reflective of emerging novel techniques in bioanalysis. This fully up to date edition includes over 30 new terms and a section of commonly used equations by bioanalysts across the field.

We would like to thank the members of the Glossary Editorial Panel for their assistance, advice and guidance and the Sponsors whose support has made this edition possible. We would also like to thank all of the Bioanalysis and Bioanalysis Zone readers, contributors and Editorial Board members for their continued support. We intend to continue to update this glossary with the inclusion of appropriate new content and timely amendments to any definition. As such, we welcome any feedback and suggestions for future editions.

Jack Lodge

Commissioning Team Manager
Taylor & Francis
Jack.Lodge@tandf.co.uk

Scope

In this glossary, 'bioanalysis' is defined as the quantitative or qualitative measurement of endogenous or exogenous analytes in biological matrices, including tissue, blood, serum, urine or other bodily fluids. The broader use of the term used by biochemists for biochemical characterization is excluded.

This glossary lists terms, definitions and equations:

- Directly associated with the field of bioanalysis;
- That describe closely related techniques, technologies and applications of bioanalysis, which are important or useful for bioanalysts to understand.

It covers:

- General bioanalytical terms;
- (Bio)analytical techniques and equipment;
- Pharmacokinetics;
- Clinical trials;
- Metabolomics;
- Antidoping testing;
- Therapeutic drug monitoring;
- Regulatory and validation terminology;
- Drug development;
- Statistical terminology.

Disclaimer and Copyright Information

Disclaimer

Whilst every effort is made by the Publisher and Editorial Board to ensure that no inaccurate or misleading data, opinions or statements appear in this glossary, they wish to make it clear that the data and opinions appearing herein are the responsibility of the contributor concerned. Accordingly, the Publisher, Editorial Board and their respective employees, officers and agents accept no liability whatsoever for the consequences of any inaccurate or misleading data, opinions or statements. Sponsors did not participate in the compilation or editing of this glossary. Sponsored terms were selected by Sponsors from the final edited list, which was compiled by the Taylor & Francis Editorial Team and the Glossary Editorial Panel.

Copyright

Terms and definitions

2D chromatography

The simplest form of multidimensional chromatography, involving two distinct chromatographic systems interfaced such that heart-cuts from the first are injected into the second. The result is combined chromatography that involves and benefits from the selectivities of both chromatographic dimensions, often with increased sensitivity as well as resolving power.

Note: See also ***heartcutting***.

3-(4-Hydroxyphenyl)propionic acid (HPPA)

A fluorogenic substrate of the enzyme horseradish peroxidase, used in ELISAs to enable higher sensitivity and extended dynamic range as compared to colorimetric detection.

abbreviated new drug application (ANDA)

Request to the US FDA for approval of a generic drug.

absolute bioavailability

Extent of unchanged drug absorbed upon extravascular administration in comparison to the dose administered intravascularly (i.e., percentage of drug absorbed unchanged).

absorption

The process, in a non-intravenous administration, whereby a drug is delivered into the bloodstream. A key dynamic function typically occurring via passive diffusion through cell membranes, and, where oral administration is involved, dominated by the small intestine. Absorption is dependent on many factors such as size, solubility and ionization behavior of a drug, and the pH, surface area and blood supply of the absorption environment.

absorption, distribution, metabolism and excretion (ADME)

An acronym commonly used in pharmacology and pharmacokinetics to reference the four key processes describing the disposition of a pharmaceutical compound.

accelerator mass spectrometry

A niche form of mass spectrometry that accelerates ions to very high kinetic energies before analysis, allowing separation of rare isotopes from more abundant isotopes. As an ultrasensitive technique, it is used to study drug metabolism and is especially suited to microdosing studies (e.g., absolute bioavailability and Phase 0 studies).

acceptance criteria

Predefined criteria, such as for accuracy or precision, used for accepting or rejecting an experimental outcome. Particularly important in regulated quantitative bioanalysis.

accuracy

The proximity of the determined value to the nominal or known true value. Percentage accuracy is calculated as (determined value/true value) × 100. Accuracy is a crucial target endpoint in quantitative bioanalysis.

accurate mass

In mass spectrometry, determination of the mass of an analyte with sufficient accuracy to enable the elemental composition to be found. Only high-resolution instruments are capable of accurate mass readings.

Note: See also ***high-resolution mass spectrometry (HRMS)***.

acid dissociation

Sample pretreatment step using a decrease in pH to dissociate an analyte from a protein (e.g., drug-antidrug antibody [ADA] complexes), often used in conjunction with various immunoassay/immunoextraction method formats to improve assay characteristics, such as an increase in tolerance of ADA detection to the presence of drug.

adverse event

Any untoward medical occurrence in a patient or clinical trial subject that has been exposed to a medicinal product, and which may or may not have a causal relationship with the treatment.

affinity

The strength of an interaction between a drug and its biological target, or more specifically the probability of a drug occupying a receptor at a given moment.

affinity-based biosensor

Device able to detect the concentration of analytes by their specific binding with several biotransducers (a biosensor component that converts biological signals into a measurable output), such as receptors, aptamers or antibodies.

AI performance monitoring

The process of continuous tracking, analysis and evaluation of an AI model to ensure it operates efficiently, accurately and reliably in real-world settings. This involves assessing various performance metrics such as accuracy, precision, recall, latency and resource utilization. Monitoring helps detect data drift, biases, anomalies or degradation in AI system performance over time.

alignment

The data processing step where one corrects for artifacts created by the analytical instrumentation, for example, chromatographic retention time (RT) variations or mass spectral shifts or shifts along the *m/z* axis between samples. Alignment is critical for many mass spectrometry-based detection methods and separation approaches, as well as nuclear magnetic resonance (NMR) data from complex samples. It must be performed to verify one-to-one correspondence between the variables being compared in order to accurately ascertain the differences in the chemical compositions between samples.

ambient ionization

Mass spectrometric analysis performed where gas-phase ions are generated under ambient conditions outside the instrument and without defined sample preparation.

analyte

A specific chemical entity being quantified or otherwise assessed, which can be an intact drug, biomolecule or its derivative, metabolite and/or degradation product in a biological matrix.

analyte fortification

Addition of the compound of interest, the analyte, to the biological matrix for preparation of calibration standard, quality control samples (QCS) or other validation samples. A common informal term is ‘spiking’.

analytical procedure

The defined sequence of steps necessary to perform a complete analysis described in adequate detail to permit the procedure to be reliably and reproducibly performed by an appropriately trained and skilled individual.

Note: See also ***method***.

analytical range

The range of concentration, or other similar measurement of abundance, of analyte in a given matrix over which the method is applicable without modification.

analytical run

A complete set of analytical and study samples including a blank sample, a zero sample, an appropriate number of calibration standards, quality control samples (QCS), and, if applicable, study samples.

anchor calibrator

A calibration standard point outside of the range of quantification, typically used to assist in fitting the nonlinear regression (e.g., 4-parameter or 5-parameter logistic) of the standard (calibration) curve in ligand-binding assays (LBA). The principle may also be justified and used in less complex and linear regression in certain circumstances.

antibody

A protein molecule generated *in vivo* in response to treatment with an antigen that is capable of binding to a specific determinant on the antigen. Also used as biotherapeutics.

antibody–drug conjugate (ADC)

Biologically active small molecule (payload) chemically linked to a monoclonal antibody (mAb).

anticoagulant

A substance added to blood during sample collection to prevent blood clotting (coagulation), e.g., heparin, EDTA, sodium citrate.

antidrug antibody (ADA)

A pre-existing or treatment-induced antibody that is capable of binding to the drug. In addition to proteins, sulfa drugs and other small molecules can induce ADAs.

Note: Also referred to as ***antitherapeutic antibody***.

antigen

A substance eliciting the formation of antibodies in a suitable host.

anti-idiotypic antibody

An antibody that binds to the idiotope of another antibody. The variable part of an antibody including the unique antigen binding site is known as the idiotype; the idiotopes are the combination of epitopes within the idiotype and are unique for each antibody. Anti-idiotypic antibodies can be generated to bind specifically to one monoclonal antibody drug.

antisense oligonucleotide

A short nucleic acid sequence that can bind to mRNA and alter protein expression.

aptamer

Nucleic acid molecule engineered to bind to various molecular targets. The mode of action of an aptamer is dependent primarily upon its tertiary structure.

aqueous normal-phase liquid chromatography (ANP-LC)

A variant of normal-phase liquid chromatography (in which the stationary phase is more polar than the mobile phase) for which the mobile phase components and additives are water-miscible. Hydrophilic interaction liquid chromatography (HILIC) and chromatography on silica hydride-based phases are popular examples of ANP-LC.

archive

Collection and storage of records (raw data, protocols, reports etc.) and specimens for a defined period of time. Typically as part of regulatory compliance and requiring security and limited access.

area under the curve (AUC)

The area under the plot of matrix (e.g., plasma) concentration of drug against time after drug administration, linked to bioavailability measurement.

artificial intelligence (AI)

The simulation of intelligence-created program machines and/or computer systems to perform tasks that require human intelligence, such as decision-making and visual perception, independent of explicit programming.

assay

Analytical method for detecting or measuring the presence, amount, state or functional activity of an analyte or other compound of interest.

assay development

The procedure of testing or measuring drug or biochemical activity within an organism or biological sample.

assay-appropriate scientific validation

One process of scientific validation where, irrespective of the stage of development in which the study is supported, assay criteria for scientific validation are defined to allow valid and documented decisions to be made from the reported concentrations.

Note: See also ***fit-for-purpose***.

atmospheric pressure chemical ionization (APCI)

A soft ionization technique that produces gas-phase ions, typically most effective for small, non-polar molecules. The process involves nebulization of a liquid sample, application of a sheath gas, and the use of a corona discharge needle with a current in the microampere (µA) range to impart charge to vaporized molecules. The resulting ions are then transferred into the vacuum interface of a mass spectrometer for analysis.

audit

A systematic and independent examination of study- or trial-related activities and documents to determine whether the activities were conducted, and the data were recorded, analyzed and accurately reported according to the standard operating procedures (SOPs), good laboratory practices (GLPs) or good clinical practices (GCPs), and other applicable regulatory requirement(s).

audit trail

An essential documented record, often automatically acquired, for an instrument, computer system or process that facilitates reconstruction of events chronologically. Typically it includes the date and time of an action, the user's name and the action(s) taken.

automation

The use of automated device(s) to replace manual steps and perform part or all of a bioanalytical procedure.

autosampler

Part of an instrument (often high-performance [or pressure] liquid chromatography [HPLC]) allowing the injection of samples in a reproducible and unattended manner. Has also been implemented with many newer immunoassay and FLOW instruments.

autosampler stability

Stability of the analyte in the processed sample under the conditions in the autosampler.

back-calculation

Process of calculating the concentrations of calibration standards according to a line best-fitted to the calibration standard responses against their nominal concentrations.

balance

A device used in a bioanalytical laboratory to weigh out solid and liquid materials, such as reference and internal standards or buffer components.

basal value

Measured value (e.g., for a biomarker) before the administration of a drug or other therapy.

baseline

The chromatographic signal of a system in the absence of an analyte or other compound monitored.

batch

A number of study samples of unknown concentration along with the appropriate standards and quality control samples (QCS) that are processed at one time.

Note: See also ***analytical run***.

bench-top stability

Stability of an analyte in a matrix during sample processing under conditions of sample handling.

between run

Period between or among several analytical or validation runs.

bias

The difference between an experimental value and a nominal value expressed as a percentage, sometimes used as a measure of accuracy or trueness.

Bias (%) = [(experimental value - nominal value)/nominal value] × 100%.

bioanalysis

The quantitative or qualitative measurement of endogenous or exogenous analytes in biological matrices, including tissue, blood, serum, urine or other body fluids.

bioassay

Analysis of the potency or strength of a substance, such as a drug, by comparing its effects on living cells or tissue *in vitro*, or living animals *in vivo*, with its effects on a standard preparation.

bioavailability

The fraction of a drug dose that reaches the systemic circulation unchanged, also indicated by the area under the curve in a pharmacokinetic plot post-administration of a drug.

biobetter

A biologic therapy that has an improved profile in terms of safety or efficacy, or both, compared to a biologic with a similar mode of action.

biocompatibility

Ability of a material to interact with a biological system appropriately without causing toxicity, a physiological reaction or immunological rejection.

biodistribution

Dispersion of a biological or medicinal compound within a biological system or organism.

bioequivalence

In the context of pharmacokinetics, this term is used in the assessment of bioavailability, including the rates of absorption and elimination after equimolar drug administration in different pharmaceutical formulations or preparations.

bioinert

Pertaining to certain materials, column components or liquid chromatography (LC) system components that are chemically designed to negate common adsorptive losses for biologic modalities. The detrimental effects on quantitative assays that are associated with the adsorptive phenomena are thus minimized or eliminated, and such columns are expected to require minimal or no passivation.

bioinformatics

The use of computational techniques to solve biological problems and develop methods and software to understand large amounts of data.

biolayer interferometry

An analytical methodology based on a shift in the interference pattern of the light reflected through a biosensor resulting from biomolecular binding on the biosensor surface.

biologic/biotherapeutic/biopharmaceutical

A diverse group of macromolecules with therapeutic potential that are usually derived from living organisms or systems and include monoclonal antibodies, proteins, peptides and oligonucleotides.

biological matrix

A material of biological origin that can be sampled for the measurement of specific analytes; matrices include blood, serum, plasma, urine, feces, cerebrospinal fluid, saliva, sputum and various tissues.

biologics license application (BLA)

Request submitted to the US FDA for approval to market a biologic drug in the US.

biomanufacturing

A field of biotechnology that focuses on using living organisms or their components to produce materials or products, typically for industrial or medical use.

biomarker

A defined characteristic that is indicative of normal biological processes, pathogenic processes or biological responses to an exposure or treatment, including therapeutic interventions.

biosensor

Protein-based receptor that is linked to a detection system and allows for the measurement of an exogenously added ligand, often a protein.

biosimilar

Biologic that is characterized as having the same amino acid sequence as an FDA-approved product with nearly identical pharmacokinetic and biological activity.

Note: Also referred to as ***follow-on biologic***.

biotransformation

Metabolic or catabolic changes to an administered drug that occur in a biological system.

bispecific therapeutic proteins

Proteins that are composed of subunits having two different antigen-binding sites, thereby binding to two different targets.

Bland–Altman plot

A statistical tool used as a measure of plotting and analyzing the agreement between two different assays. One of the ICH M10 recommended approaches when comparing methods in a cross-validation of a bioanalytical assay.

Note: Also referred to as ***difference plot***.

blank sample

A sample of a biological matrix to which no analytes and no internal standard have been added, which is used to assess the specificity of a bioanalytical method, the absence of matrix effects, and for interference testing. Sometimes also referred to as a double blank due to the absence of both types of materials where a sample that has only been spiked with internal standard may be referred to as a blank.

blood:plasma distribution ratio

The extent to which a drug is distributed between plasma and the red blood cell fractions of blood, often expressed in the blood:plasma concentration ratio of the drug.

blood–brain barrier

A semi-permeable endothelial membrane separating blood from cerebrospinal fluid, representing a barrier to the transport of cells and xenobiotics to the brain.

bottom-up proteomics

The study of the protein structure whereby the sequence is reconstructed from individually identified fragment peptides. In this approach, the samples are subjected to proteolytic digestion, typically using trypsin, and protein identification is performed by peptide sequencing with MS/MS.

Note: See also ***top-down proteomics.***

bradford assay

A dye-binding assay that uses a differential color to measure the concentration of protein in a solution.

Taylor & Francis
Taylor & Francis Group

bridging immunoassay

An immunoassay method commonly utilized for detection of antidrug antibodies (ADAs) that is enabled by the formation of a ternary complex or 'bridge' where one arm of the ADA binds to the capture reagent (e.g., solid phase adsorbed or biotin-labeled drug) and the second arm binds to the detection reagent (e.g., hapten-, enzyme- or ruthenium-labeled drug). Often the detection reagent is a labeled version of the capture reagent. An analogous assay may also be used for quantitation of analytes.

calibration curve

A set of calibration standards at various known concentrations whose measured instrument responses are used to construct a regression curve to measure concentrations of study samples and quality control samples (QCS) or incurred samples.

calibration range

The interval between the upper and lower limits of quantitation (ULOQ and LLOQ) that define the concentrations of analyte in the calibration standards (including these concentrations) for which it has been demonstrated that the analytical procedure meets the requirements for precision and accuracy.

Note: See also ***analytical range***.

calibration standard

A sample typically processed similarly to an unknown sample or quality control to which a known amount of analyte has been added to be used in a series of calibrants for a standard curve.

candidate surrogate end point

An indicator used in place of another in a clinical trial in order to determine the success of a treatment.

capacity factor

More commonly known as 'retention factor', k (previously k´) is a measure of chromatographic retention, for which the calculation involves both the retention time and the column void time. $k = (t_R - t_0)/t_0$ where t_R is retention time and t_0 is the column void time.

capillary zone electrophoresis

Method in which analytes are separated in liquid media or in a gel matrix in a narrow-bore capillary, based on differential migration due to their charge-to-size ratio. Separation is performed in a narrow-bore capillary generally filled with a buffer solution across which an electric potential is applied.

capture capability

Ability of the immobilized ligand on the surface of a plate well, bead or another surface to capture the target from the sample solution.

carrier protein

The use of a protein-based additive in order to avoid or minimize adsorptive effects originating within sample vials, plates or chromatographic columns and assemblies.

carryover

The inadvertent transfer of an analyte to a blank sample or other samples in a batch after the analysis of sample(s) containing analyte. Typically, this occurs following analysis of samples with a high analyte concentration. Most commonly this occurs in chromatographic analyses characterized by injection sequences where low-level or blank samples are injected after higher level samples.

CAR-T cell (or chimeric antigen receptor T cell)

T cell that has been engineered to express, at its extracellular surface, an artificial antigen receptor, for example, against a certain type of cancer or virus.

cell therapy

Administration of living cells to a patient for the replacement or treatment of diseased or dysfunctional cells.

cell-based neutralizing antibody assay

Method for the detection or quantitation of neutralizing antidrug antibodies (ADA) that block the functional properties of the drug. These assays utilize a cell line that is responsive to the drug either by directly responding to it or by responding to a ligand that shows altered activity in the presence of drug.

Centers for Disease Control and Prevention (CDC)

A national public health agency in the United States that is responsible for protecting and promoting public health and safety through the control and prevention of disease, injury and disability.

centrifugation

A process that involves the use of centrifugal force for the sedimentation of heterogeneous mixtures with a centrifuge. In bioanalysis, it is often used to separate blood from plasma, to separate protein precipitates from the liquid fraction, to pellet suspended cells or to separate two immiscible solvents during liquid–liquid extraction.

certificate of analysis (CoA)

A document that demonstrates the characterization of a purchased material such as a reference standard. A CoA for an analytical standard will commonly include key parameters such as purity, chemical formula, stability and number, as well as the approach by which these characteristics were measured. CoAs generated under the appropriate regulations may be used to support good laboratory practice (GLP), good clinical practice (GCP) or good manufacturing practice (GMP) studies.

chemiluminescence

A physiochemical phenomenon present in some chemical reactions in which the release of a photon occurs when an electronically excited product returns to a lower energy state.

chiral chromatography

Chromatographic technique that is capable of separating enantiomers via diastereomeric or inclusion complex formation with the bonded phase, resulting in differential partitioning into the mobile phase.

chiral compound

A compound that contains one or more asymmetric center(s).

chiral inversion

Enzyme or chemically mediated conversion of one enantiomer to its antipode (opposite enantiomer) with no other change in the molecule. This phenomenon is significant in the context of chiral drugs, as it can influence drug metabolism and efficacy.

chromatogram

In chromatographic analyses, a graphic display of chromatographic output, typically showing the response as the y-axis and time as the x-axis.

chromatographic column

Essential component of a liquid or gas chromatographic system, containing the stationary phase and through which flows the mobile phase. Separation is typically effected through partitioning, adsorptive, electrostatic or affinity-based interactions between the analyte in the mobile phase and the stationary phase.

chromatography

A system using a stationary phase and a mobile phase to effect separation of molecules in a given sample.

Note: See also ***chromatographic column***.

clinical benefit

A clinically meaningful, positive effect of an intervention, e.g., the reduction of pain, increased sense of well-being, a positive effect on how an individual functions or survives. Usually related to a bioanalytically determined drug concentration such as a steady state or trough value measured during the trial.

clinical bioanalytical sample

A sample received from a patient or healthy volunteer (e.g., from a clinical trial) for bioanalysis.

clinical laboratory improvement amendments (CLIA)

Regulates clinical laboratory diagnostic testing in the USA and requires clinical laboratories to be certificated.

clinical outcome

An outcome that defines or portrays how an individual feels, functions or survives.

clinical trial

Study to evaluate a new drug or treatment in healthy or diseased human subjects.

clinical utility

A conclusion that the use of a medical product will lead to an overall improvement in health outcome or provide valuable information about diagnosis, treatment, management or prevention of a specific disease. Clinical utility includes the potential variety of benefits or risks. This conclusion is tied to a specific drug dosing regimen, one that produces a drug blood level that gives rise to the therapeutic effect.

clinical validation

A process to establish that an instrument, tool or test acceptably identifies, measures or predicts the specific concept of interest. Validation of the bioanalytical method requires testing of accuracy and precision, drug stability, matrix effect and other parameters as directed by the EMA and/or US FDA guidances for bioanalytical method validation.

co-administered medicines

Two or more drugs administered concurrently to a subject.

coefficient of variation (CV)

A statistical term used for the measurement of precision. It is equivalent to relative standard deviation (RSD) and is calculated as standard deviation/mean, or %CV as CV × 100.

collision-induced dissociation/collision activated dissociation

A technique in mass spectrometry where molecular ions are accelerated through the application of electrical potential and allowed to collide with neutral gas molecules to facilitate their fragmentation.

comedication stability

The process of assessing the stability of an analyte in the presence of a compound that is administered to the subject together with the analyte. Such assessments have been requested by regulatory agencies when a fixed dose combination (FDC) dosage form is being administered. In these cases, the matrix stability of one drug must be determined in the presence of the other drug in the combination at a ratio indicative of the FDC.

companion diagnostic

A medical device, typically an *in vitro* diagnostic (IVD) test, that provides information that supports the safe and effective use of a corresponding drug or biological product.

competitive ligand-binding assay

An analytical methodology based on the competition of an analyte with a suitably labeled version of the analyte (sometimes involving an enzyme/substrate reaction) for a receptor or antibody. In a competitive assay the quantitative signal is due to labeled analyte species but is inversely related to the determined analyte concentration.

compliance

The adherence to standard operating procedures (SOPs), good laboratory practices (GLPs), good clinical practices (GCPs) or other regulatory standards. It is typically demonstrated through the accurate and complete record keeping of activities (e.g., sample custody and analysis) allowing for post study reconstruction and examination of the raw data and events.

computer software validation

A process of using predefined protocols and procedures to test and document the suitability and integrity of computer software for its intended use.

conjugation

See ***phase II drug metabolism***.

contamination

An occurrence in which analyte material from a known or unknown source (e.g., from another sample) accidentally enters a sample, a blank or analytical component, resulting in erroneous measurements.

context of use (COU) - biomarkers

A concise description of the specified use of a biomarker and its purpose in drug development.

contract manufacturing organization (CMO)

Independent organization that offers specific manufacturing services to other companies or parties working in the pharmaceutical, biotechnology and medical device industries on a contract basis.

contract research organization (CRO)

Independent organization that offers clinical trial and other research support services to other companies or parties working in the pharmaceutical, biotechnology and medical device industries on a contract basis.

convergence chromatography

See ***supercritical fluid chromatography (SFC).***

convolutional neural network (CNN)

A specialized deep learning model designed specifically for processing structured, grid-like data, such as images. They are widely used in computer vision tasks like image classification and object detection, and can be applied within bioanalysis to detect patterns, extract features and classify complex biological structures.

coronavirus disease (COVID-19)

An infectious respiratory disease caused by the viral strain SARS-CoV-2, which is spread via respiratory droplets and can trigger mild to severe symptoms in those affected.

counter ion

A general term used to describe an ionic species with opposite charge to the analyte, which may represent the ion used to form a salt to improve the solubility of chromatographic performance.

CRISPR

Clustered regularly interspaced short palindromic repeats (CRISPR) refers to the bacterial defence systems found in the DNA of archaea and bacteria. This can be utilized for systems that can be programmed to edit and cut DNA and genetic code by utilizing a CRISPR-associated (CAS) enzyme.

critical reagent

Essential component of an assay (particularly ligand-binding assays [LBA]) whose characteristics are crucial to assay performance. These reagents may be specific capture reagents, antibodies, peptides and conjugates, and they require thorough characterization and documentation. Critical reagents may require significant amounts of time to acquire and/or to determine if suitable for use. They are usually analyte specific, difficult to replace and have a direct impact on the results of an assay.

cross-reactivity

In immunology, cross-reactivity refers to the reaction between an antibody and an antigen that differs from the antigen (analyte) of interest. It arises when a molecule has an epitope sufficiently similar to one on the analyte of interest to cause that molecule to bind to the antibody in a ligand-binding assay (LBA) in a similar way (with similar or different affinity) to the analyte of interest. Specificity is related to the concept of cross-reactivity. If an antibody is highly specific, it has low cross-reactivity with molecules other than the analyte of interest.

cross-validation

Comparison of performance of a (developed) method with a different bioanalytical method through the analysis of the same set of samples. Cross-validation may include statistical comparisons of results for quality control and incurred samples.

cumulative urinary excretion curve

Plot of the cumulative amount of test substance excreted into urine versus time upon administration of the test substance.

curvature

Within linear regression, the manifestation of a nonlinear (i.e., curvilinear) response versus concentration profile within a given concentration range for a quantitative bioanalytical method. From a statistical approach, curvature is the rate at which the slope changes. It is the second derivative of any function; for a straight line, the second derivative is '0', for a quadratic regression model (also a linear function), the rate is positive or negative.

cut point

The value at, or above, which instrument response is considered positive and below which response is considered negative (in an antidrug antibody/immunogenicity assay).

cytochrome P450

A superfamily of heme-containing enzymes that can metabolize a variety of compounds via multiple pathways.

data card

A structured summary of relevant characteristics of a dataset that provides key information about its contents, origin, quality and intended use. It includes a descriptive section that provides details such as the number of samples, collection protocols and associated metadata. Additionally, it features a scorecard section, which offers a quantitative analysis of dataset characteristics based on applicable criteria and metrics.

data management

All disciplines relating to managing data as a valuable resource within bioanalytical laboratories. Data quality, integrity and security are the core of data management to ensure the data lifecycle is under control.

daughter ion

See ***product ion***.

deconvolution

In the context of biomolecule mass spectra, charge deconvolution is a program or algorithm that identifies peaks associated with different charge states for given molecular entities, and combines these into simplified spectra involving only mass (not *m/z*) and response. Deconvolution may also be applied to deal with peaks arising from isotopic distributions in the same kinds of molecules, in a process called deisotoping. This term is also used for the computational derivation of overlapping (co-eluting) peaks in certain chromatography-based procedures.

deep learning

A subset of machine learning that uses artificial neural networks with multiple layers ('deep') to process complex data and learn patterns. It is the driving force behind artificial intelligence (AI) advancements in fields like image recognition, natural language processing and autonomous systems.

derivatization

The chemical modification of functional groups to change the characteristics of compounds to be more favorable for analysis (e.g., more sensitive, differentiated from other molecules in the matrix, more specific, more volatile, fluorescent).

diagnostic assay

An assay appropriated to use in clinical decision-making for an individual patient. Such assays generally fall into one of six categories:

- Assays that screen for disease in an apparently healthy population;
- Assays used to aid in the diagnosis of a particular disease;
- Assays that monitor a disease or the efficacy of its treatment;
- Assays that stratify risk for a particular disease;
- Assays that prognose the natural course of a disease or condition;
- Assays that predict response to a therapeutic intervention.

Note: See also ***companion diagnostic***.

diastereoisomer

Stereoisomers of a compound, with multiple chiral centers, that have different absolute configurations at one or more, but not all, chiral centers. Such compounds have different physicochemical properties, and, in theory, can be resolved under conventional methods of chromatography.

difference plot

See *Bland–Altman plot*.

digestion

The enzymatic digestion of a macromolecule (usually protein) into smaller fragments (peptides) prior to analysis.

digital twin

A virtual representation of a physical object, system or process that continuously updates in real-time using data from sensors, simulations and analytics. It enables monitoring, analysis and optimization by mirroring real-world conditions digitally. Digital twins can support personalized medicine by providing virtual models of patients to guide clinical decisions, including treatment selection and assessments. They also enable the creation of large, diverse virtual populations for *in silico* clinical trials and contribute to quality control and process optimization in drug manufacturing.

dilution

The procedure of adding control matrix to quality control or incurred samples. This process is used to bring incurred samples with concentrations above the upper limit of quantification (ULOQ) into the calibration curve range for analysis.

dilution QC sample

Samples of control matrix spiked with analyte exceeding the upper limit of the validated concentration range, to which additional control matrix is added prior to analysis to bring sample concentration into calibration range. Used to evaluate the acceptability of incurred samples analyzed after dilution.

dilutional linearity

Demonstration that spiked quality control samples with concentrations exceeding the upper limit of the validated concentration range can be shown to give the same concentration (within acceptable accuracy and precision) when assayed at multiple dilutions to give results in the validated concentration range.

discriminative metabolomics

The process of comparing the metabolites present in multiple samples collected under different donor conditions (e.g., disease states, drug treatment), conducted to identify which metabolites are associated with different sample donor conditions.

diversion of LC flow

Typically used to direct mobile phase eluent containing contaminants or interferences, within a time window before and/or after the retention time of the analytes of interest, away from the liquid chromatography–mass spectrometry (LC–MS) source. Usually a make-up mobile phase is directed to the LC–MS source while the eluent is diverted away in order to maintain instrument stability (e.g., avoid drying the curtain plate).

doping analysis

Laboratory procedures aimed at ascertaining the use of banned performance-enhancing substances and methods in sport by the analysis of biological fluids.

dosage regimen

The systematized schedule under which drugs or drug candidates are administered for pharmacokinetic evaluation or therapy; that is, the proper mass and proper time interval between compound administration required to produce clinical efficacy or to maintain a therapeutic concentration in the body.

dose

A measured quantity of a therapeutic agent taken at one time.

dose-response curve

The graphical presentation of pharmacological response versus amount of compound administered (e.g., dose).

dosing interval

The time period between multiple administrations of a drug.

dosing vehicle

Substance or formulation within which a drug is administered: used to facilitate the absorption or administration of the drug.

dried blood spot (DBS) sampling

A matrix-sampling methodology based on applying whole blood (e.g., obtained from venous draws or a heel-, tail- or finger-prick) onto a (paper) substrate, which is subsequently dried and sealed in bags with desiccant for possible storage and shipping prior to extraction and analysis.

droplet digital PCR (ddPCR)

The third generation of polymerase chain reaction (PCR) that allows for precise quantification of low abundant nucleic acid within samples. This works by separating samples via water-in-oil emulsions to create droplets, which are then used to identify and quantify genetic material.

drug metabolism

See ***biotransformation***.

drug–drug interaction

The effect of co-administered drugs on the pharmacokinetics (PK) and pharmacodynamics (PD) of the drug of interest. This often results from competitive binding at one enzyme, transporter or receptor.

dry-down

The evaporation of solvents, from sample extracts during the sample preparation process, for the typical purpose of concentration and increasing sensitivity.

electrochemiluminescence (ECL)

An analytical methodology based on the detection of light generated during electrochemical (redox) reactions of compounds in solution or attached to an electrode surface.

electronic workflow

The technology infrastructure facilitating the automated flow of an organization's electronic content.

electrospray ionization (ESI)

A very prevalent means of generating gas-phase ions for subsequent mass spectral analysis. A soft ionization technique, an electrospray-based ion source releases pre-formed ions from the liquid phase via a process known as 'ion evaporation' into gaseous ions.

elimination half-life

After peak concentration is reached, the time necessary to reduce the drug concentration in the plasma to one-half.

elution

In chromatography, the process of desorbing or releasing an analyte from the stationary phase with a defined set of conditions involving the mobile phase.

enantiomer

One of two stereoisomers that are non-superimposable mirror images of each other.

endogenous compound

Components naturally present in biological fluids obtained from animals or humans.

endpoint

A predetermined point precisely defined to which a variable must reach in order to conclude an experiment.

enzyme

Catalytic proteins that speed up the rate of a chemical reaction or enable the conversion of one chemical to another in a living organism.

enzyme induction

The increase in the rate of enzymatic processes resulting in faster metabolism of a compound, usually caused by repeated treatments with an inducing molecule. If a drug stimulates its own metabolism, this is called autoinduction.

enzyme inhibition

The decrease in the rate of metabolism of a compound usually caused by competition for binding to an enzyme system responsible for metabolism of the compound.

enzyme-linked immunosorbent assay (ELISA)

A form of immunoassay where the enzyme is linked to a protein that can bind to a captured analyte and, through the subsequent addition of the enzyme's substrate, generate a molecule that is detected using UV, fluorescence or luminescence.

epimer

Stereoisomer with more than one chiral center that differs in the configuration at only one center.

epitope

The part or sequence of an antigen that is recognized by the immune system (i.e., antibodies, B or T cells).

esterase

A family of hydrolase enzymes that react with esters to form an acid and alcohol. Their activity commonly requires inhibition for robust quantitative analysis of ester analytes in biofluids.

European Medicines Agency (EMA)

Regulatory body responsible for the protection of public and animal health in the European Union through the scientific evaluation and supervision of use of medicines.

ex vivo

That which occurs outside a living organism.

excretion

The final elimination of a compound and its metabolites from the body's systemic circulation via the kidney into urine, *via* bile into feces and *via* the lungs into the air.

extractability

The extent to which an analyte can be recovered from a biological matrix by extraction techniques, commonly using a solvent.

extrapolation

In the context of calibration curves, the use of the characteristics of an established concentration–response relationship for a defined calibration range as a basis to predict concentrations outside the range. This process is synonymous with the method of standard addition and associated techniques to calculate endogenous levels of biomarkers in biological matrices.

false-negative

A false-negative result for a sample indicates that the sample shows a test result of 'negative' for an analyte of interest, although the analyte is actually present in the sample or is present at a concentration below the detection limit of the assay. In anti-drug antibody assays, the analyte is actually present in the sample but its response is below the cutoff point of the assay.

false-positive

A false-positive result for a sample indicates that the sample shows a test result of 'positive' for an analyte of interest, although it is not actually present in the sample. In anti-drug antibody assays, the analyte is not present in the sample but its response is above the cutoff point of the assay.

FDA Form 483

A form used by the US FDA to document and communicate concerns discovered during their inspections.

fingerprinting

A reproducible pattern expressed in the data that can be used to classify individual samples into categories using a number of multivariate and/or machine learning approaches.

first-in-human (FIH)

A clinical trial in which a medical procedure or drug candidate, previously developed and evaluated through *in vitro*, animal testing or mathematical modeling, is tested on human subjects for the first time. Commonly referred to as first-time-in-human (FTIH) or, in earlier literature, first-time-in-man (FTIM).

first-pass effect

The phenomenon where drugs may be metabolized following absorption from the gastrointestinal tract (GI) but before reaching systemic circulation. Generally, this process reduces oral bioavailability of the drug.

fit-for-purpose

A bioanalytical method that has been qualified or validated to achieve desired scientific rigor and parameters that meet the intended purpose.

Note: See also ***tiered approach***.

flow cytometry

Laser-based analytical technique used for cell counting, cell sorting and biomarker detection.

follow-on biologic

See ***biosimilar***.

Food and Drug Administration (FDA)

Agency within the US Public Health Service that is responsible for approving the safety, efficacy and marketability of medicines, among other health-related services.

formalin-fixed paraffin-embedded (FFPE) tissue specimens

A widely used method for preserving and preparing biopsy specimens for histological examination, experimental research, diagnostics and drug development. The process begins by obtaining a tissue specimen, which is then fixed in formalin to preserve proteins and cellular architecture. After fixation, the tissue is embedded in a paraffin wax block, allowing for thin sectioning and mounting onto microscopic slides for detailed examination.

formulation

Process during which an active drug is combined with different chemical substances to form the final medicinal product.

free drug

A drug in the body that is not bound to a protein (e.g., albumin), target or antibody.

free jet expansion

The diffusion model for carrier gas and ions transitioning from a mass spectrometer ion source through an orifice aperture into the vacuum region.

freeze-thaw stability

The assessment or establishment of stability of an analyte in a matrix when frozen and thawed, usually with reference to three freeze-thaw cycles in method validation.

full validation

Establishment of all validation parameters for a bioanalytical method to ensure its validity for sample analysis for each analyte in accordance with health authority regulations and industry guidelines.

functional neutralizing antibody assay

A neutralizing antibody binds to distinct functional domains of a therapeutic drug or vaccine and blocks its activity or function. A functional neutralizing antibody assay detects if an antidrug antibody (ADA) neutralizes a drug or vaccine's activity.

gas chromatography (GC)

A chromatographic technique that uses a carrier gas, typically helium or hydrogen, as a mobile phase where the injected liquid sample is vaporized in the injection port. The walls of a GC column are coated with a thin viscous liquid layer, the stationary phase, on an inert solid support. GC is often used to separate and analyze volatile and semi-volatile compounds.

gene editing

A molecular biology technique that can precisely add, delete or alter specific genes or regions of the genome.

gene therapy

A therapeutic technique that involves delivering genes or oligonucleotide sequences into cells to modify gene expression or function and treat disease.

generative AI

A type of artificial intelligence that is capable of creating new content, such as text, images, music, videos or even code, based on patterns it has learned from existing data. Unlike traditional AI, which typically analyzes and classifies existing data, generative AI can generate entirely new data that is similar to what it has been trained on. For example, in bioanalysis, generative AI can be used to design and optimize bioanalytical assays, predict biological outcomes, generate synthetic data and integrate multimodal data.

generic drug

A drug created with the same chemical structure as an existing brand-name drug, equivalent in dosage form, safety, strength, route of administration, quality and performance characteristics, which can enter the market with appropriate regulatory approval once the patent of the original drug has expired.

good clinical practice (GCP)

A standard for the design, conduct, performance, monitoring, auditing, recording, analysis and reporting of clinical trials that provides assurance that the data and reported results are credible and accurate, and that the rights, integrity and confidentiality of trial subjects are protected.

good laboratory practice (GLP)

A set of regulations that establish a framework for the planning, conduct, monitoring, documentation, reporting and archiving of laboratory studies.

good manufacturing practice (GMP)

A set of regulations that provide a structured framework for the planning, execution, monitoring, documentation, reporting and archiving of the manufacturing processes for drugs, food and active pharmaceutical ingredients.

gradient elution

A chromatographic technique where the composition of mobile phases is modulated continuously or in a stepwise manner to separate compounds within a single chromatographic run.

heartcutting

A chromatographic technique where specific chromatographic region(s) are transferred to a separate chromatographic system or dimension (generally of different selectivity) for additional separation. This is typically applied in multidimensional chromatography.

hematocrit

The volumetric proportion of red blood cells in whole blood.

hemolysis

Lysis (rupture) of red blood cells resulting in release of hemoglobin and other cellular matter into the plasma, thus changing its composition.

hepatic clearance

The degree of loss of a drug in passage through the liver, mainly through hepatic metabolism and biliary excretion. Typically measured by the hypothetical volume of distribution in millilitres of unchanged drug cleared in 1 minute via the liver.

heteroscedasticity

Non-uniform variability (or scatter) across a set of another predictor variable as pertains to instrumental response across a range of concentrations, an important reason for weighted linear regression.

high dose-hook phenomenon

See *prozone effect*.

high ionic strength dissociation assay (HISDA)

A ligand-binding assay protocol that uses high ionic strength conditions to dissociate protein–protein interactions for improved drug tolerance in antidrug antibody (ADA) assays or for reduction of target interference.

high-performance (or pressure) liquid chromatography (HPLC)

A chromatographic technique used to separate components in a mixture. A sample is injected onto a liquid mobile phase, which is pumped at high pressure through a column, packed with adsorbent material (stationary phase). Components of different affinities to the stationary phases are retained differently and resolved. It is often more simply referred to as liquid chromatography (LC).

high-resolution mass spectrometry (HRMS)

A technique capable of accurate measurement of the molecular weight of a compound via their mass-to-charge ratio (m/z). HRMS is generally referred to having a mass spectral resolving power >10,000, where resolution is m/δm (with m being mass and δm the smallest mass difference for which the two peaks m and [m+δm] are resolved).

high-throughput screening

Method by which large compound libraries are tested rapidly for activity against specific target(s) in drug discovery.

hit

Identified molecule that has the ability to bind to its target to bring about a biological response, which may require further development.

hit confirmation

Series of methods/assays applied to an identified hit molecule to confirm its structure and activity profile.

hit identification

Process to analyze molecules to discover which has activity against a target.

hit-to-lead/lead generation

Stage in early drug discovery where small-molecule hits are evaluated and undergo limited optimization to identify promising lead compounds.

homogenate

Suspension of tissue cellular fragments and constituents obtained after the tissue is homogenized, lysed, sonicated and/or digested.

homogenization

A technique used to break down tissues, which can be mechanical, sonication, bead beating and/or enzymatic.

homoscedasticity

Equal or uniform variability (or scatter) across a set of another predictor variable as pertains to instrumental response across a range of concentrations.

Hook effect

The phenomenon typically observed in one-step sandwich ELISA whereby particularly high analyte concentrations result in decreased signals, compared with lower nominal concentrations on the curve, resulting in a hook-shaped curve at the high concentration region.

hydrophilic interaction liquid chromatography (HILIC)

A variant of normal-phase chromatography that uses hydrophilic (polar) stationary phase and hydrophobic (mostly organic, typically aprotic) and water miscible mobile phase. Retention increases with hydrophilicity of analytes and the order of elution is opposite to that obtained with reversed-phase chromatography.

hydrophilic-phase extraction (HPE)

A solid-phase extraction technique specifically for highly polar and charged analytes, such as oligonucleotides, where hydrophilic interaction liquid chromatography (HILIC) is the operational mode of retention and release. HPE features an amino-bonded phase on a silica base.

hydrophobic interaction liquid chromatography (HIC)

A chromatographic technique separating molecules (e.g., proteins and peptides) based on their hydrophobic properties. The hydrophobic stationary phase binds analytes like proteins from aqueous solutions to different extents depending on the protein structures and a range of controllable factors including concentrations of salts, pH, temperature and organic solvents.

hyperlipidemia (lipemia)

Abnormally high levels of lipids and/or lipoproteins in blood, often associated with genetic factors and diabetes, as well as dietary factors. Reliable bioanalysis of hyperlipidemic samples may be compromised due to the lipid content and method performance is typically checked using several lots of spiked blank hyperlipidemic matrix.

IC_{50}

Measure of the potency of an inhibitor on its biological target, measured as the concentration of inhibitor required to reduce the target's binding ability or function by 50%, which is dependent on the concentration of the target.

ICH M10 (bioanalytical method validation and study sample analysis)

Published by the International Council for Harmonisation of Technical Requirements for Pharmaceuticals for Human Use (ICH), the ICH M10 is a guideline intended to provide recommendations for the validation of bioanalytical methods for chemical and biological drug quantification and their application in the analysis of study samples. The guideline is implemented by regulatory bodies globally, including the US FDA and European Commission. These should be regarded as minimal requirements.

immobilization capacity

Maximum amount of ligand that can be immobilized on the surface of one plate well or bead.

immunity

The state of being resistant to a specific infectious disease or pathogen; immunity may be innate (the body's natural first line of defense against harmful substances, e.g., skin, mucous membranes and other barriers), adaptive (immunity gained through infection or vaccination, which leads to the body generating an immune response against future infections of the same pathogen) or passive (immunity gained by the receipt of antibodies from an external source, e.g., a baby receiving antibodies through the placenta).

immunoaffinity chromatography

Type of liquid chromatography in which the stationary phase consists of an antibody or antibody-related reagent. The method can be used in assays for a particular target or for purification and concentration of analytes prior to further examination by another technique.

immunoaffinity liquid chromatography–mass spectrometry (IA–LC–MS)

Using a capture protein, aptamer or antibody to extract target analytes from a biological sample matrix prior to LC–MS analysis.

immunoassay

Technique that uses the specific recognition and binding of antibodies to an analyte (protein or other molecule) in order to detect or quantify the analyte.

immunocapture

Direct capture of a molecule by an antibody immobilized onto a surface.

immunocompromised

The state of having a reduced ability to fight infections and other diseases due to a weakened immune system. Immunocompromised individuals can either present a dysfunctional immune system from birth (primary immune deficiency) or inherit such immunodeficiency from another condition or medical treatment (secondary immune deficiency).

immunocytochemistry

A technique used to visualize specific proteins or antigens by binding them with fluorophore-conjugated antibodies, allowing visualization under a fluorescent microscope.

immunogen

A molecule (e.g., protein, small-molecule carrier protein conjugate) that will elicit the production of antibodies in animals and, sometimes, humans upon repeated treatments.

immunogenicity

The ability of a molecule, usually with reference to a therapeutic (e.g., protein, nucleic acid, carbohydrate, lipid or small molecule), to provoke an immune response in the body of a human or animal.

immunogenicity assay

Method to detect an immune response to an administered therapeutic (usually a protein) in biological fluids (usually serum or plasma).

immunohistochemistry (IHC)

An important application of monoclonal as well as polyclonal antibodies to determine the tissue distribution of an antigen of interest in health and disease. IHC is widely used for diagnosis of cancers; specific tumour antigens are expressed *de novo* or upregulated in certain cancers.

imprecision

Equivalent meaning to precision, pertaining to the degree of proximity or agreement of measurements within a replicate set, without reference to a nominal or true value. Usually assessed by calculating the relative standard deviation or relative standard error of the mean for replicate measurements.

in silico

Experiments performed on a computer for the purpose of the evaluation or prediction of *in vivo* results, or for the optimization of conditions to be used for planned experiments. Some important *in silico* analyses may include simulating a biologic or biochemical process, testing a predictive model under a specific set of computational parameters or performing database searches.

in situ

An action, process, observation or analysis that takes place in the natural, original position or location. In pharmacological studies of biological systems, *in situ* processes usually take place in an organism and/or organ at the specific site where a disease process or drug action is exerted.

in vitro

An action, process, observation or analysis that takes place outside living organisms, using isolated organs, cells, cell constituents or artificial culture media.

in vivo

An action, process, observation or analysis that takes place in living organisms.

inaccuracy

Numerical difference (positive or negative bias) between the mean of a set of replicate measurements and the true or nominal value.

incubation

In reference to disease, the period of time or process in which pathogens increase in number or size in the body, but no symptoms of disease are yet present. From an analytical perspective, this refers to the incubation procedure of reactants in an experiment.

incurred sample

Study sample from human or animal subjects, pre- and usually post-administration of therapeutic drugs. Study subjects may be either human, for clinical studies, or non-human, for animal studies.

incurred sample reanalysis

Repeated measurement of analyte concentration from a portion of the incurred study samples from dosed subjects to evaluate the reliability of the original results and the method itself.

in-source fragmentation

In liquid chromatography–mass spectrometry (LC–MS), fragmentation of a molecule or further fragmentation of a molecular ion in the mass spectrometer vacuum interface region between the source and low-pressure analytical segment, usually caused by collisions occurring during acceleration from the source probe electrode tip to the lens or cone at the head of the mass filter rail under reduced pressure but in the presence of nitrogen curtain or shield gas.

instrument qualification (IQ/OQ/PQ)

A process that tests the suitability of the given instrument(s) or instrument system and associated software for their intended usage following a predefined protocol:

- The instrument qualification (IQ) is normally performed during initial installation to verify and record the identity and proper set up of the test system.
- The operational qualification (OQ) is performed during validation in order to verify proper operation of the system under the testing conditions intended for analysis.
- The performance qualification (PQ) is performed during validation to confirm and record system performance figures of merit such as sensitivity, accuracy, specificity and reproducibility under analytical operating conditions.

inter-assay accuracy

Accuracy within the context of multiple analytical occasions, for example, from a mean of 18 replicates over three analytical occasions (six or more replicates on three occasions) and a corresponding nominal concentration.

inter-assay precision

Precision of the replicate measurement of an analyte between separate analytical occasions, typically measured in terms of %CV for each nominal concentration.

interference

Any substance from a sample or sample matrix that impacts the accuracy and/or precision of an analytical measurement.

interim data

Results derived from analyses performed during the course of a trial or experiment prior to their finalization.

intermediate precision

A measure of precision/agreement that reflects within-laboratory variations, for instance different days, different analysts, different equipment, among others.

internal standard

Substance(s) (e.g., a physicochemically similar analogue, or stable isotope-labeled compound) added to calibration standards, quality control samples (QCS) and study samples at a known and constant concentration to correct for experimental variability during sample preparation and analysis.

International Council for Harmonisation of Technical Requirements for Pharmaceuticals for Human Use (ICH)

Formed in 1990, the ICH brings together regulatory authorities and the pharmaceutical industry to discuss scientific and technical aspects of drug registration. It aims to achieve greater harmonization worldwide to ensure safe, effective and high-quality medicines are developed and registered in the most resource-efficient manner. It aims to achieve this through the development of harmonized guidelines that are adopted by member countries in place of local/regional guidelines (ICH guidelines).

interpolation

The means of calculating the concentrations of unknown samples based on a simple regression model from calibration standards.

intra-assay accuracy

Accuracy as it pertains to bioanalytical validation, typically from a mean of six replicates within a single analytical run as compared to a corresponding nominal concentration.

intra-assay precision

Precision as it pertains to bioanalytical validation, typically calculated as the %CV or RSE (relative standard error) from the analysis of six replicates within a single analytical run.

intravascular administration

The route of administration where the drug is directly introduced into the blood stream via a blood vessel. IV refers to intravenous administration. PO (*per os*) refers to oral administration. Combined IV and PO experiments provide pharmacokinetic calculations for oral bioavailability.

intrinsic clearance

Theoretical clearance of unbound drug on a molecular basis by an elimination organ. Typically provided from metabolism or transport molecular kinetics. Processing intrinsic clearance by an organ mathematical model provides theoretical organ clearance in a bottom-up manner.

Investigational New Drug (IND) application

The means by which researchers or pharmaceutical companies obtain permission to start a clinical trial. The US FDA reviews the IND application for safety and/or efficacy to assure that research subjects will not be subjected to unreasonable risk.

Investigator's Brochure (IB)

A compilation of the clinical and nonclinical data on the investigational product(s) with analysis and discussion that is relevant to the study of the investigational product(s) in human subjects.

ion source

A critical device of a mass spectrometer (MS) that forms gas-phase ions.

ion suppression

Reduced ionization efficiency or detector response in mass spectrometry as a result of competition for ionization between the analyte of interest and matrix or analytical components or excipients.

ion trap mass spectrometer

A mass spectrometer that traps ions in a cell or along a linear quadrupole, such that scanning ejects ions from the trap according to their *m*/*z*.

ion-exchange chromatography

Chromatographic separation mode based on manipulation of charge and electrostatic interactions between the analytes, mobile phase and stationary phase.

ion-mobility spectrometry

Technique used in conjunction with mass spectrometry to separate ions based on relative mobilities in a drift cell with an electric field and carrier buffer gas. The mobility of an ion depends on cross-sectional area, shape and charge.

ion-pairing chromatography

A chromatographic method that utilizes additives, typically in a mobile phase, that undergo electrostatic binding to oppositely charged analytes. A frequent goal of ion-pairing chromatography in reversed phase systems is to enhance retention of polar ionic analytes and to increase separation efficiency. Additional effect expected is to reduce or eliminate adverse peak shapes, caused by a positively charged analyte interacting with silanols groups on silica-based columns.

ion-pairing reagent

A mobile phase additive used in ion-pairing chromatography to selectively increase the retention and improve the peak shape of charged analytes. Typically, an ion pairing reagent contains both a hydrophobic region and an ionizable group whose charge is opposite to that of the analyte. The resulting neutral or less polar complex shows improved chromatographic properties and peak resolution.

isobaric isomers

Compounds with identical molecular formulae and molecular weights that are measured at the same *m/z* in a mass spectrometer but have different spatial configurations in a molecule.

isocratic elution

A liquid chromatographic elution using a single and constant mobile phase composition.

isotope dilution

The technique to add known amount of isotopically labeled substance chemically identical to the analyte to ensure monitoring or tracing of the analyte. The use of isotopically labeled internal standard is one form of this technique. The ratio of the dilution of the isotopically enriched substance can then be used to determine the amount of analyte in the sample.

isotopologue

An isotopically labeled, or isotopically distinct, analogue of a given compound.

kinetics

The rate(s) of change in chemical and biochemical reactions, or the branch of science that observes such changes in a physical, chemical or biological system.

kosmotropes

Solutes that are very water-soluble, very hydrated through hydrogen bonding, and that order the structure of water. Trehalose (the disaccharide mycose) is a familiar kosmotrope used in research and commerce. Kosmotropes can be considered as solutes with an anti-chaotropic effect.

lab-on-a-chip

See *microfluidics*.

laboratory information management system (LIMS)

Software package utilized in (bio)analytical laboratories as a central database for sample management, analysis and produced data.

large language model (LLM)

A type of artificial intelligence (AI) that is trained on large amounts of text data to understand, generate and manipulate human language. These models are built using deep learning techniques, particularly a type of neural network architecture called transformers, which allows them to process and generate text efficiently and accurately.

lead candidate

A compound or molecule that has been selected through pharmaceutical discovery screening procedures because it shows appropriate target selectivity and potency, has a strong therapeutic potential and justifies further development.

lead optimization

The drug discovery process entailing specific chemical modification of lead compounds, designed to enhance their safety, potency, selectivity, pharmacokinetic or absorption, distribution, metabolism, excretion and toxicity (ADMET) properties, with the goal of producing a viable drug candidate, suitable for formal development.

least squares

A statistical method of determining a regression equation that best describes the relationship between two variables, based on the minimal sum of the squares between data points and regression.

ligand-binding assay (LBA)

Qualitative or quantitative method based on the binding of ligand molecules to targets (drugs, antibodies or other biological molecules), typically used for biomolecules where the reliance is on highly specific epitope–paratope interactions between antigen and antibody.

limit of detection (LOD)

The lowest concentration of an analyte that a bioanalytical procedure can reliably differentiate from background noise (e.g., 'detected and not quantified').

linear regression

An approach for modeling the linear relationship by regression, which is the method to minimize errors in the y-axis dimension. In bioanalysis, this is used to describe the linear relationship between analyte concentration and instrument response (typically the ratio between analyte and internal standard).

lipidomics

A comprehensive measure of all the lipophilic species detectable in a given sample, typically employing liquid chromatography coupled to tandem mass spectrometry and high-resolution mass spectrometry.

liposomal drug

A drug formulation consisting of phospholipid molecules that enclose a water droplet in which the drug is located. Administration of an active compound in such a formulation may alter its biopharmaceutical properties.

liquid chromatography (LC)

Chromatographic technique that employs a liquid mobile phase, injection of a liquid sample, and a packed-column stationary phase of appropriate chemistry for the desired selectivity. This technique can be coupled to a variety of detectors, most notably mass spectrometry, for bioanalysis.

liquid–liquid extraction

Sample extraction that relies on the partitioning of an analyte between an aqueous component and a water-immiscible organic component. Partitioning may be optimized by alteration of solution conditions including pH, temperature, salt concentration and buffer additives.

locked nucleic acid (LNA)

Oligonucleotide containing one or more of the 2′-O,4′-C-methylene-β-D-ribofuranosyl nucleosides, called LNA monomers. The major feature of LNAs is the high-affinity hybridization to complementary nucleic acids because of high thermo-stability, resulting in enhanced selectivity and assay sensitivity.

long-term stability

Assessment of the analytical recovery of an analyte in its natural matrix following extended periods of (usually) frozen storage compared to its initial state prior to storage.

lower limit of quantification (LLOQ)

The lowest amount of analyte in a sample that can be quantitatively determined with predefined precision and accuracy.

luciferase

The generic term for a class of oxidative enzymes that produce bioluminescence. Luciferase is the enzyme in an enzyme–substrate pair, in which the substrate is termed luciferin. Luciferases occur naturally in organisms such as the firefly and are also widely used in biotechnology for bioluminescence imaging microscopy and reporter genes. Applications are similar to those of fluorescent proteins, but unlike fluorescent proteins, luciferases do not require an external light source.

luciferin

The generic term for a class of light-emitting organic compounds present in organisms that produce bioluminescence. Luciferin is the substrate in an enzyme–substrate pair, in which the enzyme luciferase causes the oxidation of luciferin, producing light.

luminometer (or luminescence microplate reader)

An instrument that measures weak emissions of visible light from a sample. The luminometer uses a photomultiplier tube and is able to measure samples as little as a few microliters, such as a sample from a well of a microplate.

machine learning (ML)

A subset of artificial intelligence (AI) in which computers learn from data to make predictions or decisions without being explicitly programmed. It uses algorithms to identify patterns in data and improve over time as more data is provided.

mass accuracy

Expressed in ppm, mass accuracy is the degree of closeness of the measured *m/z* value to the actual *m/z* value. Calculated by mass error/actual mass-to-charge $\times 10^6$, where mass error is the measured *m/z* value - actual *m/z* value ((measured mass - actual mass)/actual mass) $\times 10^6$.

mass resolution

Resolution needed to separate two mass spectral peaks, $m/\Delta m$, where m denotes m/z and Δm denotes difference in m/z, to typically 5% above baseline.

mass spectrometry

Analysis of proteins and other molecules involving ionization and measurement of the mass-to-charge ratio of the resulting ions, enabling the identification of molecules in pure samples and complex mixtures.

mass-to-charge (*m/z*)

The characteristic of a molecule or molecular fragment that represents its nominal mass divided by the number of charges the molecule carries. This value is typically fragment ions in mass spectrometry assays and is used to define the nominal mass settings for the filtering of the analyte out of the mixture of all present ions.

master schedule

A GLP requirement for all nonclinical laboratory studies conducted at the testing facility indexed by test article and containing the test system, nature of study, date the study was initiated, current status of each study, the identity of the sponsor and name of the study director.

matching matrix

Blank biological matrix or surrogate matrix prepared from a recipe, used for the preparation of calibration standard and quality control samples (QCS), intentionally similar to the matrix of (incurred) samples requiring analysis. Matrix matching is often used in analysis of biological fluids or tissue where blank tissue is unavailable or limited to best compensate for matrix effects. Given that the matrix can vary sample-to-sample and patient-to-patient in a clinical trial, it is not possible to unambiguously match the matrix in all respects.

matrix

The natural or intrinsic complex environment in which a desired analyte is measured, such as whole blood, plasma, serum, urine, cerebrospinal fluid or other biological samples. A matrix not containing exogenous chemicals (except those required for sample collection or storage, such as an anticoagulant) and their metabolites is called a blank matrix.

matrix effect

The direct or indirect alteration in assay response (including both sample preparation and analysis) due to the presence of matrix constituents in extracted samples.

matrix factor (MF)

The ratio of the analyte response in the presence of matrix to the response in the absence of matrix. MF = analyte response in the presence of matrix/analyte response in the absence of matrix.

matrix-assisted laser desorption/ionization (MALDI)

A soft ionization technique used in mass spectrometry, allowing the analysis of drugs, biomolecules and large organic molecules. It works through a three-step process that involves mixing the sample with a suitable matrix material, using a laser to trigger ablation and desorption and finally ionizing the molecules in the hot plume of ablated gases, which are then accelerated into the mass spectrometer.

maximum tolerated dose (MTD)

Within the context of preclinical toxicology, an MTD study is a high dose used in chronic toxicity testing that is expected on the basis of an adequate subchronic study to produce limited toxicity when administered for the duration of the test period.

mechanism of action (MOA)

A term used to describe how a drug or other substance produces an effect in the body. A drug's MOA could be how it affects a specific target in a cell, such as an enzyme, or a cell function, such as cell growth. Knowing the MOA of a drug may help provide information about the safety of the drug and how it affects the body. It may also help identify the right dose of a drug and which patients are most likely to respond to treatment.

Medicines and Healthcare products Regulatory Agency (MHRA)

UK agency responsible for ensuring that medicinal products and medical devices are both effective and acceptably safe.

metabolite

A product of metabolism; in bioanalysis, this usually refers to a product of the endogenous metabolism, but metabolites can also be products of metabolism of an administered therapeutic or other exogenous substances.

metabolite features

Peaks with a unique mass-to-charge ratio or deconvoluted as a cluster of different mass spectrometry species (adducts, neutral losses) corresponding to a unique *m/z*, a unique retention time and with an intensity value (or area under the peak).

metabolite profiling

The measurement of all low-molecular-weight metabolites and their intermediates in a biological system.

Note: See also ***metabolomics***.

metabolites in safety testing (MIST)

The detection, confirmation and comparison of the exposure of drug metabolites observed in human clinical trials with those observed in animal studies. Used to establish the safety of the human metabolites through demonstrating adequate exposure in animal species.

metabolome coverage

The ability of an analytical technique to detect a subset of all metabolites (endogenous or exogenous) in complex biological samples. No single technology can currently provide the overall analysis of all analytes in such samples and, as a result, a combination of techniques is required to obtain a holistic metabolome coverage.

metabolomic biomarker

An endogenous metabolite whose concentration changes in response to disease or the treatment thereof. Such metabolites can be used for the purpose of diagnosis, disease subcategorization, prognostication and prediction of therapeutic sensitivity to treatments.

metabolomics

Often used interchangeably with the term 'metabonomics', this is an analytical approach that entails the comprehensive analysis of the low-molecular-weight compounds (<1000 Da) involved in the metabolic networks of living organisms and their response to pathophysiological or other stimuli. This methodology involves the use of advanced metabolite profiling techniques, such as nuclear magnetic resonance (NMR) spectroscopy and/or mass spectrometry linked or not with a separation technique such as gas chromatography (GC), liquid chromatography (LC) or capillary electrophoresis (CE).

meta-metabolomics

Quantitative analysis of metabolite patterns in a complex host–microbiome system (including multiple partners); for example, used to identify metabolic networks related to health or disease issues.

method

Comprehensive description of all procedures used in sample analysis.

method development

A process to develop and define the sample preparation procedure and liquid chromatography–mass spectrometry (LC–MS) condition, so that the method is sensitive, precise and reproducible.

method qualification

Subset of the method optimization processes that verifies method performance to demonstrate that an analytical method is working according to predefined acceptance criteria.

method transfer

An agreed process or protocol between two laboratories in order to ensure specific analytical practices can be reproduced and deliver comparable results in each laboratory location.

method validation

A comprehensive set of documented experiments to investigate whether an analytical method is functioning according to predefined acceptance criteria. For regulated bioanalysis, criteria should be in compliance with guidelines published by regulatory authorities.

micellar electrokinetic chromatography

Separation technique hybrid of electrophoresis and chromatography where a surfactant, generally ionic (e.g., sodium dodecyl sulfate [SDS]), is added to the separation buffer at a higher concentration than its critical micelle concentration (CMC). During migration micelles act as a pseudo-stationary phase allowing solute partition through both hydrophobic and electrostatic interactions and simultaneously to electrophoretic separation.

micelle

An aggregate of molecules in a colloidal solution, forming as a result of hydrophobic and hydrophilic regions on the molecular structure. For example, a liposomal suspension.

microbore column

A chromatographic column with an inner diameter comprising between 1 and 2.1 mm and operated at mobile phase flow rates typically between 50 and 1000 µl/min. This configuration leads to increased detection sensitivity and it is attractive for the analysis of low-volume (or low-concentration) samples.

micro-elution

In the context of solid phase extraction (SPE), the media and associated procedures that feature lower sorbent weight and specialized design compared to traditional SPE, ultimately allowing reduced elution volumes and typical avoidance of evaporation steps while maintaining recovery and performance.

microflow

Liquid chromatography employing a mobile phase with a relatively low flow rate compared to conventional techniques, typically 1–50 µl/min, and with appropriate miniaturized construction and operation.

microfluidics

A field of technology using systems in which very small volumes of fluids are handled. For bioanalysis, this term usually refers to miniaturized devices that contain small flow channels and that combine one or multiple analytical functions in a single device.

Note: Also referred to as *lab-on-a-chip*.

microsample

Sample of blood or any other biological matrix in the low µl/µg range utilized for certain preclinical or clinical studies. The sample may be liquid or dried, as in a dried blood spot.

microsampling

The process of collecting and analyzing minute samples, no more than 10–20 µl. This term normally refers to blood samples.

miniature mass spectrometer

Use of a special reduced-size mass spectrometer, allowing for use outside of the traditional laboratory setting.

minimal residual disease (MRD)

Pertaining to the small number of cancer cells that remain in the body after cancer treatment is complete, and which cannot be detected.

minimum required dilution

In ligand-binding assays, a minimum extent of dilution necessary to bring the assay into a range of concentration-response linearity, or sufficiently reduce any background signal interference in the analysis.

mixed-mode

The use of multiple retentive modes to affect a separation, pertaining to a chromatographic or solid-phase extraction process. For example, ion-exchange can be performed in conjunction with reversed-phase partitioning.

mobile phase

In chromatography, the mobile phase is a solvent (liquid, gas, supercritical fluid) that moves through or along the stationary phase of a column, resulting in the distinct chromatographic migration of solutes.

molecular ion

Produced by loss or gain of one or more electrons from a neutral molecule starting point. These are either positive ions or negative ions.

molecularly imprinted polymer (MIP)

An artificial affinity material consisting of a synthetic polymer, formed in the presence of a compound (the template), that is later removed and, thus, leaves specific binding sites or a cavity for the template and structurally related molecules.

monitoring peptide

In protein liquid chromatography–mass spectrometry (LC–MS) bioanalysis, a term used to describe a unique peptide derived from the proteolytic digestion of a specific protein analyte, but one that is different from the surrogate or signature peptide. The signal from the monitoring peptide(s) is normally given as a ratio to that of the surrogate peptide for a given sample, and variations in this could be reflective of the stability of the protein analyte *in vivo*. In specific cases there may be more than one monitoring peptide for a given protein analyte.

monoclonal

Pertaining to a specific protein from a single clone of cells, all molecules of this protein being the same.

monoclonal antibody

Antibody produced by cloned cells derived from a single lymphocyte. Distinct from polyclonal antibodies, which are heterogeneous.

monolith

A solid support that consists of a single piece of porous material characterized by a bimodal pore size distribution (macroporous and mesoporous), which confers favorable mass transfer properties, a large surface area and low pressure drops, and is suitable for use in analytical or purification methods.

mRNA vaccines

A form of vaccination that uses a copy of messenger RNA (mRNA) to elicit an immunological response. An mRNA vaccine eliminates the need for the use of a bacteria or virus for the creation of a vaccine.

multi ascending dose (MAD)

A format of dosing in which a drug is administered repeatedly at intervals shorter than those required to completely eliminate the drug from the previously given dose. This form of dosing is used to study the pharmacokinetics (PK)/pharmacodynamics (PD) of multiple doses for safety and tolerability. The dose is increased over time to a predetermined maximal level.

Note: Also referred to as ***multiple ascending dose***.

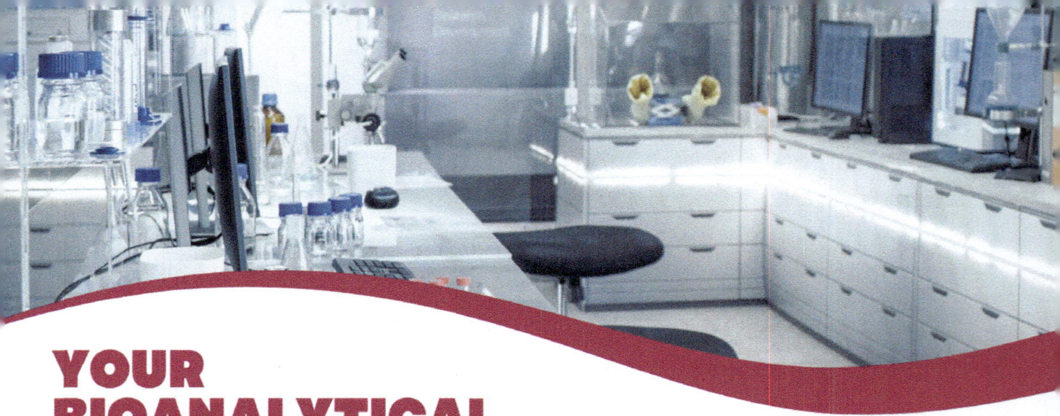

multi-analyte

Pertains to a methodology focused on more than one analyte, each of which will be subject to appropriate acceptance criteria in a quantitative assay.

multiple heartcutting 2D separation

In this mode of 2D-LC separation, several selected regions of the first separative dimension are selected for further resolution by transferring the fluid exiting the first separation during several short (e.g., a few seconds to about a minute) intervals to the second separation column for further separation of sample constituents that were not initially separated by the first column.

multiple reaction monitoring (MRM)

A quantification strategy generally used in triple quadrupole (QqQ) mass spectrometers, in which an analyte ion with a particular mass-to-charge ratio (the precursor ion), most often corresponding to the intact ion of a target analyte, is selected by a first quadrupole (Q1) in the mass spectrometer. The precursor ions are then subjected to a collision-induced dissociation reaction with neutral gas, resulting in the formation of product ions, each with a particular mass-to-charge ratio, which are selected in another quadrupole (Q3) and subsequently detected.

multiplexing

The ability of an analytical technique or device to process or analyze multiple analytes in a sample in parallel. This term also refers to the determination of multiple analytes using the same assay or run.

multiply-charged ion

An ion of more than one charge, with each charge situated on a different ionizable moiety on a given molecule. It is common in large molecule ionization such as a peptide, oligonucleotide and protein.

multi-site study

Any study that has phases conducted at more than one site.

nanoflow

Nanoliter per minute flow rates employed in chromatographic separations with very narrow-bore capillary columns (≤500 nm i.d.).

nanoflow liquid chromatography

A liquid chromatographic system or method employing mobile phase flow at flow rates in the order of nanoliters per minute (nl/min).

nanoscience

The study, management and manufacturing of matter on a nanometer scale. A nanometer equates to one millionth of a millimeter and is the scale used to measure atoms and molecules.

neutralizing antibody (NAb)

An antibody that is formed *in vivo* in response to treatment with an antigen and that binds to a drug and blocks its function. For an enzyme drug, a neutralizing antibody would block its action on the substrate. For an agonist or antagonist drug, an antibody that blocks the drug binding to its ligand would neutralize the drug. Antibodies that bind to epitopes on a drug that do not affect the function of the drug are non-neutralizing antidrug antibodies.

New Drug Application (NDA)

A process in the USA through which drug sponsors formally apply for approval by the US FDA for the sale and marketing of a new pharmaceutical.

nominal concentration

Theoretical concentration notation, used in the preparation of calibration standards and quality control samples.

non-cell-based neutralizing antibody (NAb) assay

An analytical technique used to assess the presence of neutralizing antidrug antibodies in a sample without using intact cells for analysis. Typically, such an assay uses the isolated drug target coated onto a plate and generates an analytical response upon binding of the drug to its target. The presence of a neutralizing antidrug antibody will interfere with the ability of the drug to bind to its target, resulting in a measurable change in assay signal.

nonspecific adsorption/binding

Undesired adsorption of analytes to the surfaces of containers or assay components, potentially leading to analyte loss or assay interference. This can be minimized by optimizing solvent composition or by using vessels with different materials or surface treatments. In immunoassays, nonspecific binding refers to the attachment of proteins other than the target to the assay plate, causing interference or artificially elevated recovery of the target analyte.

nontargeted analysis

Analysis of a complex sample without predefined selection criteria, aiming to identify previously unknown components. This contrasts with targeted analysis, which focuses on specific, predefined analytes.

non-zero calibrator

A calibrator that contains a known, non-zero concentration of analyte. In chromatography-based assays, the internal standard (IS) is added to these calibrators. In immunoassays, a non-zero calibrator refers to a calibration point containing a known concentration of the calibration protein.

normal-phase chromatography

A chromatographic mode using a polar stationary phase (e.g., native silica) and a nonpolar mobile phase. Hydrophilic analytes interact strongly with the stationary phase and elute later, while lipophilic analytes elute earlier due to weaker interactions.

novel isoelectric target depletion (ITaD)

An approach to specifically deplete targets based on their biophysical properties to reduce their interference in assays.

nuclear magnetic resonance (NMR) spectroscopy

An analytical technique that utilizes the magnetic properties of certain atomic nuclei to elucidate the physical and chemical properties of the atoms or molecules that contain them. NMR provides detailed structural information and can be used for both quantitative and qualitative analyses.

oligonucleotide

A strand of DNA or RNA, typically containing less than 30 nucleotide units.

online extraction

A bioanalytical technique that integrates sample extraction (often solid-phase extraction) directly with chromatographic analysis, allowing biological samples such as plasma to be processed with minimal pre-treatment.

optimization

The process of systematically varying analytical method parameters to identify the optimal conditions for a specific application. This process can be guided by Design of Experiments (DoE) methodologies.

oral administration

A route of drug or substance administration via the mouth, including swallowing (*per os*), as well as buccal, sublingual and prelingual routes.

Organisation for Economic Co-operation and Development (OECD)

An international organization of 34 countries, established in 1961, that promotes economic progress and world trade. The OECD issues Good Laboratory Practice (GLP) guidelines that are followed by many countries, including those in Europe.

origin-adjusted approach

In quantifying biomarkers or endogenous compounds by liquid chromatography-mass spectrometry (LC-MS), this approach involves spiking authentic matrix with known amounts of non-labeled analyte to generate a calibration curve, which is then mathematically adjusted to pass through the origin, effectively correcting for endogenous analyte levels. Sample concentrations are interpolated from this adjusted curve.

orthogonal

Refers to two or more separation or detection modes for an analytical method that provide uncorrelated selectivities for analytes. Combining orthogonal methods (e.g., different chromatographic or mass spectrometric techniques) enhances overall separation and identification capability.

out of specification (OOS) investigation

A documented process initiated when a laboratory result or outcome falls outside of predefined acceptance limits. The investigation identifies the root cause, assesses potential impact and implements corrective and preventive actions.

outlier

A data point that deviates markedly from other observations in a data set, potentially indicating an error or anomaly. Statistical methods can be used to identify and assess outliers.

over-curve concentration

A sample with an analyte concentration exceeding the upper limit of quantitation (ULOQ) of a validated analytical method.

oxidation

A chemical reaction in which an atom, ion or molecule loses electrons, or its oxidation state increases. Often involves an increase in the number of bonds between carbon atoms and more electronegative atoms, such as oxygen, or a decrease in the number of bonds between carbon atoms and less electronegative atoms, such as hydrogen.

pandemic

An outbreak of an infectious disease that rapidly spreads across multiple countries or continents. The most recent example is the COVID-19 pandemic, caused by Severe Acute Respiratory Syndrome Coronavirus 2 (SARS-CoV-2).

parallel reaction monitoring (PRM)

A targeted mass spectrometry technique in which the third quadrupole is replaced with a high-resolution mass analyzer, enabling simultaneous detection of all target product ions in a single analysis.

parallelism

A condition in which the dose–response (or dilution–response) curve of a test sample is parallel to that of the calibration standard curve. In immunoassays and bioassays this is typically assessed by comparing the responses of serially diluted samples containing endogenous analyte to the standard curve. The goal is to detect matrix effects or differences in antibody binding affinity between endogenous and standard analyte. Successful parallelism indicates that dilution of the test sample does not introduce bias in analyte quantification and the test sample behaves as a true dilution of the standard.

parallel-line analysis (PLA)

A statistical method for the comparison of potency between a reference product and test product. It is used to calculate relative potency by comparing the dose–response curves of the two products.

paratope

The specific region of an antibody that recognizes and binds to an epitope on an antigen. It is located at the tip of the antibody's variable region and is formed by six complementarity-determining regions (CDRs) from both the heavy and light chains.

Note: Also referred to as ***antigen-binding site***.

parent ion

See ***precursor ion***.

partial least-squares (PLS) regression

A statistical method used to model relationships between two matrices (predictors and responses), especially when predictors are highly collinear or when there are more variables than observations. PLS projects both predictor and response variables into a new space that maximizes their covariance, making it especially useful in chemometrics and omics data analysis. Extensions, such as orthogonal PLS (O-PLS) and O2-PLS, further refine this approach for various applications, such as for metabolomic data.

partial validation

A series of analytical experiments performed to confirm the reliability of a previously fully validated bioanalytical method after a modification (e.g., change in matrix, instrument or procedure) or transfer. The extent of partial validation depends on the nature and significance of the modification.

passivation

Pertaining to the accumulation through sequential injections, on a chromatographic column or system, of biologic material that occupies adsorptive sites on these components, subsequently and eventually allowing the full sensitivity of a chromatographic assay to be manifest.

patient stratification

The process of dividing a patient population into distinct subgroups based on specific characteristics, such as disease features, biomarkers or predicted response to therapy, often used to enable tailored treatment strategies.

peak area

The area under a chromatographic peak, measured from the baseline, which is proportional to the amount (concentration or mass) of the analyte present in the sample, depending on the detector used.

peak area ratio

The ratio of the chromatographic peak area of the analyte of interest to that of an internal standard, used to correct for variability in sample preparation and analysis.

peak capacity

A measure of chromatographic separation efficiency, defined as the maximum number of peaks that can be theoretically baseline-resolved within a given chromatographic run or time window. Higher peak capacity indicates better separation of complex mixtures.

peak fronting

A type of chromatographic peak asymmetry where the leading edge (front) of the peak is broader or more sloped than the trailing edge. It is often caused by column overload, poor column packing or incompatible solvent composition, resulting in some analyte molecules eluting earlier than expected.

peak height

The maximum vertical distance from the baseline to the apex of a chromatographic peak, which is proportional to the amount (concentration or mass) of analyte, depending on the detector and analysis conditions.

peak height ratio

The ratio of the peak height of the analyte of interest to the peak height of an internal standard in a chromatogram, used to normalize for analytical variability.

peak tailing

Distortion of the chromatographic peak shape where the trailing edge (tail) is broader than the leading edge, deviating from the ideal Gaussian profile. Causes include secondary interactions with the stationary phase, column degradation, inadequate sample clean-up or suboptimal pH conditions.

peak tailing factor

Quantifies the asymmetry of a chromatographic peak. It is calculated using the widths of the front and back of the peak at a specified percentage of peak height, commonly 5% or 10%. A value greater than 1 indicates tailing, while a value less than 1 indicates fronting.

Note: Also referred to as *symmetry factor.*

PEGylated lipid nanoparticle

Coating the surface of nanoparticles with polyethylene glycol (PEG), or "PEGylation", is a commonly used approach for improving the efficiency of drug and gene delivery to target cells and tissues. Various strategies to coat and characterize nanoparticles with PEG have established important trends in PEG size, shape, density, loading level, molecular weight, charge and purification.

per aqueous liquid chromatography

Chromatographic mode that is a variant of reversed-phase chromatography, typically performed on unmodified silica using highly aqueous (80–100%) mobile phases. It exploits surface siloxane groups and highly energetic adsorption sites on silica to achieve separation.

percent difference from theoretical

See *bias*.

peripheral blood mononuclear cell (PBMC)

Any peripheral blood cell having a round nucleus. These cells consist of lymphocytes (T cells, B cells, NK cells) and monocytes, whereas erythrocytes and platelets have no nuclei, and granulocytes (neutrophils, basophils and eosinophils) have multi-lobed nuclei. In humans, lymphocytes make up the majority of the PBMC population, followed by monocytes and only a small percentage of dendritic cells.

peripheral compartment

The sum of all body regions to which a drug eventually distributes, but are less perfused and therefore are not in instantaneous equilibrium with the concentration in blood or plasma.

personalized medicine

An emerging practice of medicine that uses an individual's genetic profile to guide decisions made in regard to the prevention, diagnosis and treatment of disease. Knowledge of a patient's genetic profile can help doctors select the proper medication or therapy and administer it using the proper dose or regimen. Personalized medicine is being advanced through data from the Human Genome Project.

pharmacodynamics (PD)

The relationship between drug concentration at the site of action (receptor) and pharmacologic response, including biochemical and physiologic effects that influence the interaction of the drug with the receptor.

pharmacogenomics

The use of genetic information to analyze a person's response to a drug. Pharmacogenomics can influence the clinical decision of which drug is best suited to an individual based on their gene variations and the suggested dosage for a specific individual.

pharmacokinetics (PK)

The kinetics of drug absorption, distribution, metabolism and elimination (ADME). Distribution occurs not only to site of action, but to multiple other tissues in the body.

pharmacology

The study of how drugs affect living systems, including how they are absorbed, distributed, metabolized and excreted. It is a bridge science that combines biology, chemistry and other disciplines.

pharmacometabonomics/pharmacometabolomics

Analysis of endogenous metabolites (aka biomarkers) in bodily fluids used to predict or evaluate the metabolism of pharmaceutical drugs, and to understand the pharmacokinetic profile of a drug. Alternatively, it is applied to measure metabolite levels following the administration of a pharmaceutical drug, to monitor the effects of the compound on certain biochemical pathways.

phase I drug metabolism

Reduction, oxidation or hydrolysis reactions, which add or expose polar functional groups (e.g., -OH, $-NH_2$, -SH) and serve to transform lipophilic drugs into more polar molecules.

Phase I trial

The first-in-human clinical trial phase to evaluate the safety and toxicity of a new treatment.

phase II drug metabolism

Metabolism that involves adding hydrophilic groups to drugs or their phase I metabolites to increase their water solubility and facilitate excretion. This is achieved through enzymes like glucuronosyltransferases and sulfotransferases. The goal is to produce more polar, less active metabolites that can be easily eliminated by the body.

Note: Also referred to as ***conjugation***.

Phase II trial

A clinical trial evaluating the efficacy and safety of a new treatment. It can be divided into Phase IIa and Phase IIb to evaluate a drug's dosing requirements and clinical efficacy, respectively.

Phase III trial

A clinical trial to evaluate the efficacy and safety of a new treatment in a large number of patients and to compare it to the current standard-of-care treatment.

Phase IV trial

A post-authorization clinical trial involving many patients to determine any rare or long-term adverse effects of a treatment.

phosphatase

An enzyme that removes a phosphate group from a molecule. This process, called dephosphorylation, is essential for cellular regulation and signaling. Phosphatases work in conjunction with enzymes called kinases, which add phosphate groups to molecules, allowing cells to finely tune protein activity and regulate various cellular processes.

phosphodiester

An inter-nucleotide linkage formed when the acidic hydroxyl group on the phosphate moiety attached to the 5' carbon on a nucleotide sugar unit undergoes a condensation reaction with the hydroxyl group on the 3' carbon on the sugar of the adjacent nucleotide.

phospholipids

A class of lipids that are the major components of cell membrane bilayers. In bioanalysis, without optimized sample clean-up, these have been identified as one of the major endogenous components that can cause matrix effects in electrospray ionization (ESI).

phosphorothioate

Inter-nucleotide bonds are similar to a phosphodiester linkage except that a sulfur atom replaces non-bridging oxygen. Phosphorothioates bestow enhanced nuclease tolerance and thus are valuable in therapeutic oligonucleotide design.

phosphorylation

The process of adding a phosphate group to a molecule, usually a protein. This addition of a phosphate group can alter the molecule's activity, shape or interactions with other molecules.

pipette

A manual or automated mechanical device that can accurately and repeatedly transfer liquid volumes of biological fluids, stock solutions and solvents.

pKa

The negative base ten logarithm of the acid dissociation constant of a compound in aqueous solution. This gives a convenient measurement of acidity or basicity with regard to the conjugate acid of a base.

placebo

A substance containing no medication and prescribed or given to humans or animals in clinical or preclinical trials as a control treatment.

plasma

The pale yellow liquid component of blood that holds the blood cells in suspension. Plasma is prepared by removing red blood cells from whole blood in the presence of anticoagulant (e.g., EDTA or heparin).

plasma protein binding

The extent to which a drug binds to endogenous plasma proteins, often expressed as the fraction of the drug that is protein bound (in percentage). Only the unbound fraction of the drug can exert pharmacological effects, and only this fraction can undergo metabolism in the liver and other tissues.

plate reader

A laboratory instrument used to measure and analyze samples in microtiter plates, which are essentially multi-well plates. It detects various biological, chemical or physical events within these samples, such as absorbance, fluorescence or luminescence.

Note: Also referred to as ***microplate reader***.

point-of-care testing (POCT)

Bioanalytical testing near or at the site of patient care (i.e., as close as possible to the patient). It is an alternative diagnostic approach to laboratory analysis.

Note: Also referred to as ***bedside testing*** or ***near-patient testing***.

polyclonal antibodies

A mixture of antibodies that are secreted by different B cell lineages. These antibodies are actually a collection of immunoglobulin molecules that react against a specific antigen, each identifying a different epitope on an antigen.

polyethylene glycol (PEG)

Any of a series of polymers $H(OCH_2CH_2)_nOH$ where n is greater than three that vary from viscous liquids to waxy solids and are used in medical and biotechnological applications. In particular, a series of water-soluble oligomers and polymers extends a biological half-life.

polymerase chain reaction (PCR)

A molecular biological method used to enzymatically amplify a single or few copies of a particular DNA sequence using short DNA sequences called DNA primers (i.e., a laboratory technique for rapidly producing thousands or millions of copies of a specific segment of DNA). It is a common tool used in medical and biological research labs to diagnose certain infectious diseases and genetic changes.

population-specific cut point

A threshold level determined for and applied to a target population to define the presence or absence of a response.

positive control

A useful proof to show that the system, reactants and the environment under which the experiment takes place are functioning without errors. Positive controls are frequently antibodies reactive to the therapeutic and are used to support immunogenicity assays.

post-column infusion

Technique for the evaluation of matrix effect profiles in liquid chromatography–mass spectrometry (LC–MS) analysis, by injection of a solvent blank or matrix blank into the chromatography column while simultaneously infusing analyte by a syringe pump to the column effluent before the detection device. It can be used to qualitatively identify regions of ion suppression or enhancement in a particular matrix extract, applied only during a method development or validation.

post-market surveillance

Identification and collection of information on the safety of a medicinal product or device following release on the market.

post-translational modification (PTM)

Chemical modification to polypeptides, that changes the properties of a protein by proteolytic cleavage and adding a modifying functional group (e.g., acetyl, phosphoryl, glycosyl and methyl) as the covalent attachment to one or more amino acids, during their biosynthesis, but after their translation from the mRNA sequence.

precipitation and acid dissociation (PandA)

An immunoassay technique that employs precipitation and acid dissociation to mitigate drug interference in immunogenicity assays.

precision

The closeness of agreement between indications or measured quantity values obtained by replicate measurements on the same or similar objects under specified (controlled) conditions. Precision as such is not quantified but refers to how repeatable a measurement can be, i.e., it is a measure of consistency. Precision is inherently related to the standard deviation of the repeated measurements, but standard deviation is a measure of dispersion, which is the inverse of precision. Standard deviation is a quantitative concept and is therefore convenient in practice. Using precision as a synonym for standard deviation should be avoided.

Three levels are distinguished by the most important validation guidelines:

- Repeatability
- Intermediate precision
- Reproducibility

precision medicine

An approach to healthcare that considers individual differences in genes, environment and lifestyle when making decisions about disease prevention, diagnosis and treatment. Instead of a "one-size-fits-all" approach, precision medicine aims to tailor interventions to specific individuals or groups of people based on their unique characteristics.

Note: Also referred to as ***personalized medicine***.

preclinical study

Studies that take place before any testing in humans. They involve evaluating a medicinal product *in vitro* (in animal or human cells/ tissues) and/or *in vivo* (in animals) to determine whether a drug, procedure or treatment will likely be helpful and safe in humans.

precursor ion

In mass spectrometry, an electrically charged molecular moiety may dissociate to form fragments, one or more of which may be electrically charged and one or more may form neutral species. The electrically charged molecular ions can be manipulated and transported from the ion source to the detector or to a collision cell to generate fragments/product ions using electric and/or magnetic fields. The electrically charged molecular ion generates fragmentation/product ions spontaneously or induced by collisions with inert gases such as Ar, He or N_2. The parent ion formation depends on the molecule's chemical structure and the solvent system's pH employed for the chromatography or dissolving of the compound.

Note: Also referred to as ***parent ion***.

predictive metabolomics

Prediction of the functional value of a treatment by means of multivariate analysis using metabolome data (biomarker/metabolite signatures) as the explanatory variable.

pre-digestion liquid chromatography–mass spectrometry with immunocapture (PrD-LC–MS IC)

A bioanalytical method where the analyte protein is first purified from the source matrix by an immunoaffinity method followed by proteolytic digestion using trypsin or another specific protease then by liquid chromatography–mass spectrometry (LC-MS/MS) analysis of surrogate peptide. This method type uses no immuno- or affinity enrichment of the surrogate peptide. In specific cases mass spectrometry (MS) methods other than tandem mass spectrometry (MS/MS) may be applied. MS seamlessly integrates with ion chromatography (IC) or liquid chromatography (LC) systems for detection and quantitation of ions using IC-MS.

pre-digestion liquid chromatography–mass spectrometry with immunocapture and selective capture (PrD-LC–MS IC SC)

A bioanalytical method where the analyte protein is purified from the source matrix by an immunoaffinity method then digested using trypsin or another specific protease followed by immunoaffinity enrichment of the surrogate peptide from the digest then quantitative analysis of the surrogate peptide by liquid chromatography–mass spectrometry (LC-MS/MS). In specific cases mass spectrometry (MS) methods other than tandem mass spectrometry (MS/MS) may be applied.

pre-digestion liquid chromatography-mass spectrometry with selective capture (PrD-LC-MS SC)

A bioanalytical method where matrix containing the analyte protein is directly digested using trypsin or another specific protease, followed by immunopurification of the surrogate peptide in the digest then by quantitative analysis of the purified surrogate peptide by liquid chromatography-mass spectrometry (LC-MS/MS). In specific cases mass spectrometry (MS) methods other than tandem mass spectrometry (MS/MS) may be applied.

pre-dose sample

A biological sample (e.g., plasma or serum) that is collected from the test subjects (per the study protocol and/or study consent forms) before they receive the study drug(s).

preventative maintenance (PM)

The regular and routine maintenance of equipment and assets to keep them running according to specifications and to prevent any costly, unplanned downtime from unexpected equipment failure. Often, a standard operating procedure (SOP) or vendor specifications, and the nature of applications (Good Laboratory Practice vs non-Good Laboratory Practice) will determine the frequency of PMs.

principal components analysis (PCA)

A statistical procedure using an orthogonal transformation of multivariate data, mainly used for exploratory analyses. It extracts and displays systematic variations and reveals strong patterns in datasets. PCA is a statistical technique for reducing the dimensionality of a dataset. This is accomplished by linearly transforming the data into a new coordinate system where (most of) the variation in the data can be described with fewer dimensions than the initial data.

principal investigator (PI)

The individual who takes direct responsibility for the completion of a funded project, directing the research and reporting directly to the funding agency and/or client/customer. The PI also oversees a clinical trial or a scientific research grant. The PI prepares and carries out the clinical trial protocol (plan for the study) or research paid for by the grant and reports directly to the funding agency and/or client/customer.

processed sample

The final extract (before instrumental analysis) of a sample that has been subjected to various manipulations (e.g., extraction, dilution, concentration).

processing batch

A group of unknown samples from study subjects, calibrators and a set of quality control samples (QCS) that are subjected to the analytical methodology together.

prodrug

A pharmacologically inactive medication or compound that is metabolized into a pharmacologically active form in the body after administration. Instead of administering a drug directly, a corresponding prodrug can be used to improve how the drug is absorbed, distributed, metabolized and excreted (ADME).

product ion

The ion that results from a charged molecular species in a tandem mass spectrometer that passes through the primary mass filter (Q1) and is then fragmented in the instrument's collision cell. The fragment/product ions can be generated spontaneously or induced by collisions with inert gases such as Ar, He or N_2.

Note: Also referred to as ***daughter ion***.

protease

An enzyme that breaks down proteins into smaller polypeptides or amino acids. Proteases are essential for many biological processes, including digestion, cell growth and immune function.

protein binding

Compound binding, with typical reference to xenobiotics, to large plasma proteins such as albumin. In the body, the extent of a drug's protein binding varies according to the drug's chemistry and certain disease states, and only the unbound fraction is considered to be freely able to move into tissues or have activity at cellular surface receptors. When aiming to analyze the unbound fraction, *ex vivo* parameters such as temperature and pH also need to be controlled.

protein precipitation

A process of removing proteins from sample matrices involving aggregation and precipitation of proteins by adding a solvent or reagent, often using an organic solvent, strongly acidic solution or concentrated salt solution.

protein quantification

The process of determining the concentration or amount of protein in a sample. This is a crucial step in various research and analytical procedures, including protein purification, sample preparation for electrophoresis and analyzing protein composition. Several methods exist, ranging from simple absorbance measurements to more complex techniques such as mass spectrometry.

protein therapeutics

Proteins that are manufactured for therapeutic use, e.g., recombinant proteins, antibody-based drugs, Fc-fusion proteins, blood factors, hormones and enzymes. Examples of therapeutics include drug therapy, medical devices, nutrition therapy and stem-cell therapies.

proteolysis

The process of breaking down proteins into smaller peptides or amino acids via enzyme activity. It is a vital cellular function that occurs in animals, plants and bacteria.

proteolytic digestion liquid chromatography–mass spectrometry (PrD-LC–MS)

A bioanalytical method where analyte proteins are quantified using the liquid chromatography–mass spectrometry (LC–MS/MS) signal from a surrogate peptide after proteolytic digestion of the sample using trypsin or another specific protease; 'reagent free' methods use no immuno- or affinity enrichment of either protein analyte or surrogate peptide. In specific cases mass spectrometry (MS) methods other than tandem mass spectrometry (MS/MS) may be applied.

proteomics

Large-scale experimental analysis of proteins and proteomes, the latter of which represent an organism's entire set of proteins. It provides a comprehensive view of protein expression, modification and activity, offering insights beyond what can be gained from studying individual proteins.

protocol

A document that describes the objective(s), design, methodology, statistical considerations and organization of a trial or a study. The protocol usually also provides the background and rationale for the trial, but these could be provided in other protocol-referenced documents.

protocol amendment

Any significant change in the design of a protocol (such as the addition or elimination of a control group). For example, the addition of a new test or procedure intended to improve monitoring for, or reduce the risk of, a side effect or adverse event; or elimination of a test intended to monitor safety, followed by documentation of the intended change to the study plan.

protocol deviation

Documentation of an unintended departure from the study plan after the study initiation date.

proxy matrix

A suitable matrix that can be used instead of an original matrix when the original matrix is available in limited amounts. It may serve as a surrogate matrix when studying, for example, matrix effects and/or endogenous biological matrix components such as transporter biomarkers.

prozone effect

False-negative or false-low results in immunological reactions due to an excess of either antigens or antibodies. Thus, an effect detected when increasing analyte concentrations results in either no change or decreased detector response compared with the preceding lower analyte concentration. This effect is often related to a detector being saturated with the analyte concentration.

Note: Also referred to as ***high dose-hook phenomenon***.

qualified assay

An assay for which not all guidance-recommended validation assessments are performed, or the extent of such assessments are limited, but which is deemed suitable (scientifically sound) in performance for the purpose of the studies it is used to support.

quality assurance

All those planned and systematic actions that are established to ensure that the trial is performed and the data are generated, documented (recorded) and reported in compliance with the applicable regulatory requirement(s). May also refer to the independent quality unit required within good laboratory practices (GLP) for quality oversight.

quality control

Selected activities undertaken within the quality management system to verify that operational activities and derived data have been verified.

quality control (QC) sample

A sample spiked with a known quantity of analyte, typically in the same matrix as the unknown samples that are used to monitor the performance of a bioanalytical method and to assess the integrity and validity of the results of the unknown samples analyzed in an individual run.

quantification range

The range of concentrations, including the upper limit of quantification (ULOQ) and the lower limit of quantification (LLOQ), which can be reliably and reproducibly quantified through the use of a concentration–response relationship.

radioimmunoassay (RIA)

A sensitive, competitive immunoassay technique whereby a limited amount of radiolabeled antigen competes with unlabeled antigen for binding to a limited amount of specific antibody. Competition with increasing amounts of unlabeled antigen provides a calibration curve from which concentrations of antigen in study samples may be interpolated.

raw data

Per the Organisation for Economic Co-operation and Development (OECD) good laboratory practice (GLP) regulations, all original test facility records and documentation, or verified copies thereof, which are the result of the original observations and activities in a study. According to the US FDA, any laboratory worksheets, records, memoranda and notes, or exact copies thereof, that are the result of original observations and activities of a nonclinical laboratory study and are necessary for the reconstruction and evaluation of the report of that study. In the event that exact transcripts of raw data have been prepared (e.g., tapes that have been transcribed verbatim, dated and verified accurate by signature), the actual copy or exact transcript may be substituted for the original source as raw data.

reactive metabolite

Drugs are generally converted to biologically inactive forms and eliminated from the body, principally by hepatic metabolism. However, certain drugs undergo biotransformation to reactive metabolites that can interfere with cellular functions. These are often electrophilic and can interact with DNA and proteins to form covalently bound products.

reagent

A substance or compound added to a system to cause a chemical reaction or to test whether a reaction occurs. Reagents are often used to indicate the presence of another substance. Common examples of bioanalytical reagents include binding reagents, such as binding proteins, antibodies and conjugated antibodies.

reanalysis

Repetition of a series of analytical procedures, from the processing step onward, on samples that have been previously analyzed.

receptor occupancy (RO)

The binding profile of therapeutic drugs to their targets on the cell surface. Typically, these drugs are antibody-based therapeutics that target specific receptors to modulate downstream signaling.

recovery (extraction)

The extraction efficiency of an analytical process, reported as a percentage of the known amount of an analyte carried through the sample extraction and processing steps of the method.

reference standard

A well-characterized substance used to spike calibration standards and quality control (QC) samples in a method, accompanied by a certificate of analysis (CoA) that provides the purity and expiration (or retest) date.

regulated bioanalysis

Bioanalysis conducted in compliance with regulatory requirements (e.g., US FDA, EMA, ANVISA or MHLW).

regulatory validation

The conduct and reporting of experimental testing of a method to demonstrate that the generated data are scientifically accurate and reproducible, to allow valid decision-making for the intended purpose of the study and comply with regulated bioanalytical standards as defined in guidance and guidelines.

reintegration

Reanalysis of the chromatographic peak.

relative bioavailability

The bioavailability of a formulation of a drug compared with that of an alternative formulation.

relative error

The difference between an estimate of a quantity and its true value. This difference (positive or negative) may be expressed either in the units in which the quantity is measured or as a percentage of the true value.

relative standard deviation (RSD)

See ***coefficient of variation***.

repeatability

The precision under the same operating conditions over a short interval of time. Repeatability is also synonymous with intra-assay precision.

reproducibility

The precision between multiple measurements of a sample or sample sets, which may include those between laboratories i.e., collaborative studies, usually applied to standardization of methodology.

resolution

A value that allows the user to evaluate the extent of separation of two or more compounds using a given technique, such as chromatography, electrophoresis or mass spectrometry.

response function

A mathematical function that adequately describes the relationship between instrument response (e.g., peak area or height ratio) and the concentration (amount) of analyte in the sample. Response function is defined within a given range.

retention time (RT)

The time taken for an analyte to reach the detector after injection and retention through a chromatographic column.

reversed-phase chromatography

A type of chromatography employing a nonpolar stationary phase and a polar mobile phase. Hydrophilic analytes have limited affinity for the stationary phase and are eluted first, while lipophilic analytes tend to adsorb to the stationary phase and are eluted by decreasing the polarity of the mobile phase.

ribonucleic acid (RNA)

A nucleic acid found in every living cell that is structurally similar to DNA. It is typically single stranded and is comprised of four ribonucleotide bases: adenine, cytosine, guanine and uracil. RNA is an essential molecule for gene coding, regulation and expression.

risk-based approach

An approach that has multiple meanings in drug development, all relating to the evaluation of the risk of failure versus the resource investment required to maintain the required quality level. The regulatory guidance and white papers by health authority authors support a risk-based approach for companies designing their own tiered testing schemes (i.e., fit-for-purpose bioanalytical strategy). It is also used in terms of a tiered approach for metabolite analyses and in consideration of biomarker analyses.

robustness

A measure of an analytical procedure's capacity to remain unaffected by small but deliberate variations in method parameters. Provides an indication of its reliability during normal usage.

r-squared

A term, often referred to as the determination coefficient, used to assess the fitness of a relationship when performing regression.

ruggedness

A measure of reproducibility of test results under normal, expected operational conditions from irregular, extraneous influences on operational parameters.

salting out assisted liquid–liquid extraction (SALLE)

The extractive process by which a solution is supersaturated with salt to cause the formation of a biphasic system between a water sample and a water miscible sample. Analytes partition between the two phases, and typically the organic phase, is taken for analysis.

sample

A generic term encompassing calibrators, controls, blanks, unknowns and processed samples.

Note: See also ***specimen***.

sample analysis

A series of analytical procedures from sample processing and/or dilution to measurement on an analytical instrument, used to determine the concentration of the test article in biological samples derived from animals or humans subjects enrolled in nonclinical or clinical studies.

sample diluent

Aqueous or organic fluids used to dilute the analyte prior to the analytical process (e.g., chromatographic separation, derivatization, binding to a receptor or antibody).

sample pretreatment

A process whereby fluid or tissue samples are homogenized, lysed, digested, sonicated, pulverized or diluted prior to analysis.

scientific validation

To provide concentration data that are scientifically accurate, reproducible and traceable to allow valid decision-making for the intended purpose of the study and that can withstand independent review (and, although not following regulated guideline 'standard operating procedure [SOP]', also review from regulators if so required). Within scientific validation, the following tiers can be defined: 'stage-appropriate scientific validation' or 'assay-appropriate scientific validation'. Sometimes referred to as 'fit-for-purpose' validation.

selected reaction monitoring (SRM)

The most selective tandem quadrupole operating mode and well adapted for quantitative applications. Precursor ions are isolated and collision-activated dissociation of the precursor occurs, with product ion isolation completing the process.

selectivity

The ability of the bioanalytical method to measure and differentiate the analytes in the presence of components that may be expected to be present. These components are generally structurally related to the analyte and could include metabolites, impurities, degradants or matrix components.

sensitivity

The lowest analyte concentration that can be measured above the noise with acceptable accuracy and precision (i.e., lower limit of quantification [LLOQ]). An alternative and statistical definition is the slope of the concentration-response calibration curve at any given point on the curve.

serum

The liquid that is obtained after clotting of the blood and subsequent centrifugation.

shotgun proteomics

Identification of proteins in the sample based on a preliminary enzymatic digestion of the mixture followed by high-performance liquid chromatography–tandem mass spectrometry (HPLC–MS/MS) characterization of the resulting peptides.

side effect

Any adverse consequence resulting from the use of a medicinal product.

signal-to-noise ratio (S/N)

The ratio of actual response signal to the differentiated background signal for a given detector.

significant human metabolite

A metabolite seen in humans that is either greater than 10% of all drug-related material in circulation or a metabolite whose exposure in humans is greater than that seen in animal species. A significant human metabolite typically requires additional monitoring or studies to demonstrate its safety.

Simoa® bead technology

An immunoassay platform which utilizes paramagnetic particles coupled with antibodies designed to bind to specific proteins and nucleic acids, allowing detection at very low concentrations.

single-dose administration

Administration of a single dose of drug by the selected route.

size-exclusion chromatography

Chromatographic separation mode based on the relative sizes of the analytes.

solid-phase analytical derivatization

A technique whereby analytes are derivatized while being retained on solid phase analytical extraction support.

solid-phase extraction (SPE)

A sample preparation procedure using packed solid sorbent and a defined protocol of conditioning, equilibration, sample pretreatment, loading and elution to provide a separation of analytes from other biological components.

solubility

The propensity for an analyte to dissolve in a liquid forming a homogeneous solution, dependent on the physical and chemical properties of the solute and solvent.

specificity

The ability to measure the analyte unequivocally in the presence of other compounds, either exogenous or endogenous, in the matrix. For International Union of Pure and Applied Chemistry, specificity is the ultimate of selectivity.

specimen

A specifically selected proportion of a material taken from a dynamic system and assumed to be representative of the parent material at the time it is taken.

Note: See also ***sample***.

Spike

(noun)

A volume of solution containing reference item added to analytical matrix to obtain a known concentration in samples such as calibration standards and quality controls.

(verb)

The action of fortifying analytical matrix with a known concentration and volume of a reference item solution.

spike recovery

The amount of analyte that is measured upon analysis of a sample (e.g., matrix) to which a known amount of analyte has been added.

Note: See also ***recovery***.

stability

The chemical stability of an analyte in a given matrix under specific conditions for given time intervals.

stable-labeled isotope

Analyte in which a few atoms are exchanged with heavy isotope counterparts, typically ^{2}H, ^{15}N or ^{13}C. It is commonly used as an internal standard in liquid chromatography–mass spectrometry (LC–MS) bioanalysis as it has very similar physical and chemical properties to the analyte and works well to compensate for the variability due to extraction, chromatography and mass spectrometry detection.

stable-labeled protein

A full-length protein in which specific amino acids are exchanged with heavy isotope counterparts. It is used as an internal standard for liquid chromatography–mass spectrometry (LC–MS) absolute quantification of protein(s) as it mimics the biochemical behaviour of the protein analyte, thus correcting for variability occurring during sample preparation, sample digestion and LC–MS detection.

stage-appropriate scientific validation

One process of scientific validation where, depending on the stage of development in which the study is supported, the proposed assay criteria for scientific validation may be different. In all stages, however, the reported concentrations support valid and documented decisions in the study. When a compound progresses in development, the study could change from nonpivotal (internal decision) to pivotal. Regulatory validation can be considered as the ultimate level of stage-appropriate scientific validation.

standard curve

The relationship between the experimental response values and the analytical concentrations of the calibrants. The term may also refer to the physical samples used to generate experimental responses and with quality controls to determine the validity.

Note: Also referred to as ***calibration curve***.

standard operating procedure (SOP)

Document that describes the recurring operations relevant to the quality of an activity that enables proper, consistent execution of the operations by someone knowledgeable in the field.

stationary phase

In chromatographic methods of analysis, typically a solid material (often modified silica or polymeric material), usually contained in a column, through which a mobile phase is moving. Separation of a mixture of analytes is achieved by differences in partitioning, adsorptive, electrostatic or affinity-type interactions between the mobile and stationary phases.

steady state

The level of the drug in blood and tissue upon multiple dosing when input and output are at equilibrium during sequential dosing intervals.

stock solution

A solution containing analyte of interest at a relatively high known concentration that can be further diluted to prepare calibration standards and quality control samples (QCS) in biological fluids.

study director

An individual holding overall responsibility for the technical conduct of the study, as well as for the interpretation, analysis, documentation and reporting of results, and represents the single point of study control. This includes approval of the study plan and its amendments, approval of the final report, and ensuring that all applicable principles of good laboratory practice (GLP) are followed.

study monitor

An individual responsible for overseeing the progress of a clinical study, and for ensuring that it is conducted, recorded and reported in accordance with the protocol, standard operating procedure (SOP), good clinical practice (GCP) and applicable regulatory requirement(s).

study plan

A document to describe the purpose and procedure of an experiment or a study. A study plan may supersede standard operating procedure (SOP) requirements.

study sample

Sample from a subject or patient registered in a study. Study subjects may either be human, for clinical studies, or non-human, for preclinical and safety studies.

supercritical fluid chromatography (SFC)

A chromatographic technique that employs a supercritical fluid as the mobile phase.

Note: Also referred to as ***convergence chromatography***.

superficially porous (core-shell) particle technology

In liquid chromatography columns, the use of particles that have a nonporous core but fully porous outer layer.

supernatant

The liquid layer resting above a lower layer or solid residue, such as after centrifugation following protein precipitation from plasma.

supported-liquid extraction

Sample extraction technique analogous to liquid-liquid extraction but with a different protocol that involves sample application to a solid support, composed of modified diatomaceous earth, and from which the analytes are subsequently eluted with water-immiscible organic solvent.

surface plasmon resonance (SPR)

A label-free optical detection technique that measures changes in refractive index at a metal-dielectric interface to monitor biomolecular interactions in real-time, enabling quantitative analysis of binding kinetics and affinities between biological molecules without the need for fluorescent or radioactive tags.

surrogate analyte

A compound analogous to the analyte of interest used to evaluate extraction efficiency and matrix effects (e.g., stable-labeled isotope analogs).

surrogate matrix

Alternative matrix used in bioanalysis in place of an endogenous matrix that is difficult to sample, recreate or maintain.

surrogate peptide

In protein liquid chromatography-mass spectrometry (LC-MS) bioanalysis, the preferred term used to describe the unique peptide derived from the proteolytic digestion of a specific protein analyte, which is then used to quantify the protein by LC-MS/MS. Other terms, such as target peptide and analytical peptide, have been used to describe this type of peptide. In specific cases mass spectrometry (MS) methods other than MS/MS may be applied.

surrogate standards

Analytes that are chemically similar to the analyte of interest. Surrogate standards are added to a sample of known concentration to determine sample processing efficiency. The role of surrogate standards is to ensure accurate quantification of analytes especially when dealing with endogenous substances or when direct measurement is challenging due to matrix interferences.

symmetry factor

See *peak tailing factor*.

system priming

Injection of extracted biological samples into a high-performance liquid chromatography (HPLC) system prior to the run under the chromatographic condition for the analytical run. System priming is mainly for blocking active sites that may adversely adsorb the analytes of interest. It should not be confused with system suitability.

system suitability

Determination of instrument performance (e.g., sensitivity, chromatographic retention and resolution) by analysis of specific samples conducted prior to submission of the analytical run.

tandem mass spectrometry

Mass spectrometry employing two analytical stages, typically separated in space (e.g., triple quadrupole or quadrupole-time of flight) or separated in time (e.g., 3D ion trap).

tandem quadrupole mass spectrometry

A quantitative tandem mass spectrometer consists of two quadrupole mass spectrometers in series, with a (non-mass-resolving) radiofrequency (RF)-only quadrupole between them to act as a cell for collision-induced dissociation. The first (Q1) and third (Q3) quadrupoles serve as mass filters. Precursor ions selected in Q1 are dissociated in the collision cell in the presence of an inert gas such as Ar, He or N_2. Resulting fragments are passed through to Q3 where they may be filtered or scanned. This configuration is sometimes referred to as a triple quad mass spectrometry and is often abbreviated QqQ.

target

Biological molecule or process with which a drug (or compound) is assumed to interact.

target candidate

Biological molecule or process with a strong therapeutic potential, for which the activity and specificity of chemical entities have been optimized.

target engagement (TE)

The interaction of a drug or lead compound with their target biomolecules such as a protein, enzyme, or receptor. Understanding TE allows research teams to evaluate whether a drug interacts with the intended target, assess compound efficacy and confirm the mechanism of action of a drug.

target validation

Process to identify and assess whether a molecular target is likely to have therapeutic benefit.

targeted analysis

Analysis of the composition of a complex sample by applying predefined selection criteria with the aim to quantify or verify the occurrence of previously identified sample components.

targeted proteomics

A mass spectrometry-based protein quantification method to test specific hypotheses for a subset of proteins, in contrast with other mass spectrometry approaches, i.e., screening proteomics, in which thousands of proteins can be identified or quantified without any prior knowledge.

targeted quantitation

Quantitation experiments to determine the protein and/or peptide levels of known targets in biological samples.

therapeutic drug monitoring (TDM)

Clinical monitoring of patient drug concentrations in plasma, serum or blood in order to enhance treatment efficacy or reduce toxicity. Typically used to treat patients taking marketed drugs with a narrow therapeutic range (i.e., those that can be easily under- or over-dosed).

tiered approach

A science-driven, fit-for-purpose strategy for scientific validation applying a predefined appropriate level of bioanalytical quality for the analysis of biological samples originating from preclinical and clinical studies. Level of pre- or in-study validation, acceptance criteria and documentation depend on the intended use of the concentration data, and consider the type of study and/or the stage of drug development in which the study data are generated.

time-of-flight mass spectrometry (TOF-MS)

Mass analyzer that utilizes a field-free vacuum chamber to separate ions by their velocity (i.e., heavier ions of the same charge reach lower speeds). The time-of-flight is then converted into the accurate mass/charge ratio of the observed ion.

tissue distribution

The extent of penetration of the administered agent into various tissues of the body.

top-down proteomics

Identification or quantification of proteins in mixtures without prior proteolytic digestion into corresponding peptides.

Note: See also ***bottom-up proteomics***.

total drug

The sum of the bound and free drug within a biological system.

total error

The sum of the absolute value of the errors in accuracy (%) and precision (%). Total error is reported as percent (%) error.

total ion chromatogram (TIC)

A graph that displays the total ion current (TIC) detected by a mass spectrometer over the course of a chromatography experiment with mass detection selectivity in the data. It shows the relative abundance of ions detected at different retention times and monitors a very large window, often of several hundred mass-to-charge units.

toxicity

Ability of a compound to cause harm to an organism.

transcription

The first stage in gene expression; the process by which DNA is copied to mRNA to facilitate protein synthesis.

translational research

The process by which the results of research performed in the laboratory are used to develop new ways to diagnose and treat disease.

turbulent flow

A liquid chromatography separation technique using narrow-diameter columns packed with large particles to create higher linear velocities and turbulence. Larger compounds will separate from smaller compounds owing to the ability of smaller compounds to diffuse into stationary phase particle pores.

ultra-high-performance liquid chromatography (UHPLC)

A liquid chromatography separation technique using support particles that often have diameters less than 2 μm in size. These smaller particles make it possible to obtain more efficient separations but also increase the pressure that is required to apply the mobile phase through a given length of column.

undersampling

For 2D liquid chromatography, this describes the transfer of portions of fluid exiting the first dimension column to the second separation column at a rate that is too slow to maintain the integrity of the first dimension separation prior to the sampling process. That is, when these transfers are made too infrequently, we say that the first separation is undersampled, which results in remixing of sample constituents that had already been resolved by the first separation column.

unknown

A biological sample that is the subject of the analysis with the goal to determine analyte(s) concentrations.

upper limit of quantification (ULOQ)

The highest concentration calibration standard of an analyte that can be quantitatively determined with pre-defined precision and accuracy, and represents the concentration above which incurred samples must be diluted to achieve a response within the calibrated range of the assay.

vaccine

A biological substance administered to stimulate immunity to an infectious disease or pathogen without inducing disease. A vaccine is typically prepared from an inactivated or weakened form of the causative agent, or from its constituents or products. Alternatively, mRNA vaccines utilize a copy of messenger RNA to stimulate an immune response.

validation

Process of gathering evidence in order to establish whether a process, standard operating procedure, piece of equipment or environment is suitable to produce a product that consistently and reliably fulfils its intended purpose, quality attributes and characteristics, according to the predetermined specification.

validation report

A summary of the experimental validation findings that define the performance characteristics of an assay for its intended use. It describes the statistical acceptance of the method.

vector

A particle used to artificially carry a foreign nucleic sequence into a cell for the purpose of replication and expression. Examples include plasmids, viral vectors and artificial chromosomes.

very-high-pressure liquid chromatography (VHPLC)

See ***ultra-high-performance liquid chromatography (UHPLC)***.

virus

A microscopic infectious agent which utilizes a host's cellular machinery to replicate. Viruses are composed of DNA or RNA surrounded by a protein coat.

volumetric absorptive microsampling

Process for the collection of a fixed, precise volume of blood using an absorbent material and subsequent storage and processing as a dried sample.

weighting factor

In linear regression, a weighting factor can be applied to correct for a situation where the variance in response varies across the fixed concentrations of calibration standards. The weighting factor gives more weight to responses with smaller variance.

white paper

Authoritative report or guide helping readers understand an issue, solve a problem or make a decision. Typically written by a panel of subject matter experts to ensure a broad consensus.

whole blood

Unmodified or unseparated blood sample typically combined with an anticoagulant. May be drawn from arteries or veins.

within-run

In validation statistics, refers to the calculation of precision and accuracy for multiple analyses of the same concentration of sample within one continuous analytical run of samples.

World Health Organization (WHO)

A specialized agency of the United Nations that is responsible for promoting and protecting global public health.

zero calibrator

Blank sample to which the internal standard (IS) is added.

Equations

absolute bioavailability

$$F = \frac{AUC_{non-IV} \times Dose_{IV}}{AUC_{IV} \times Dose_{non-IV}}$$

where:

- AUC = area under the plasma concentration–time curve
- Dose = administered dose of the drug
- IV = intravenous administration
- non-IV = any other administration route (e.g., oral, subcutaneous)

chromatographic resolution (R_s)

$R_s = (\sqrt{N}/4)*((\alpha-1)/\alpha)*(k_2/(1+k_2))$

where:

- R_s = chromatographic resolution
- N = theoretical plate count
- α = selectivity, the ratio k_2/k_1
- k_2 = retention factor of the later eluting peak
- k_1 = retention factor of the earlier eluting peak

fraction unbound (F_u)

$F_u = C_u/C_{tot} = 1 - F_b = 1 - C_b/C_{tot} = 1 - C_b / (C_b + C_u)$

where:

- F_b = fraction bound
- C_b = bound compound concentration, the portion of the compound in plasma that is bound to proteins and therefore not freely available for pharmacological action. This is the fraction that remains in the original plasma after equilibrium dialysis
- C_{tot} = total concentration of compound in plasma
- C_u = free (unbound) compound concentration, the portion of the compound in plasma that is not bound to proteins. This is the concentration measured in the protein-free dialysate after equilibrium dialysis

matrix effects

Internal standard (IS) normalized matrix effect = mean of (peak area ratio in presence of matrix, where both analyte and internal standard are added to extracts of control matrix)/(peak area ratio of analyte and internal standard in absence of matrix)

Note: A ratio of means is different from a mean of ratios.

$$\%\text{bias} = \frac{\text{mean measured conc.} - \text{nominal conc.}}{\text{nominal conc.}} \times 100$$

$$\%\text{CV} = \frac{\text{standard deviation (SD)}}{\text{mean measured conc.}} \times 100$$

%Recovery = 100 × mean peak area ratio (extracted samples containing analyte to which internal standard is added post-extraction)/peak area ratio (post-extraction-spiked samples, where both analyte and internal standard are added to extracts of control matrix)

measurement bias

The tendency of a measurement to over-or under- estimate the true (nominal) value of a population parameter.

Bias (%) = ([experimental value - nominal value]/nominal value) × 100

% receptor occupancy (RO)

$$\%RO = \frac{\text{drug bound receptor conc.}}{\text{total receptor conc.}} \times 100\%$$

theoretical plates

N, the number of theoretical plates, is a parameter used to evaluate the efficiency of a chromatographic column. It reflects the column's ability to minimize peak broadening and maximize separation. A higher number of theoretical plates indicates better column performance and sharper, more defined peaks. It may be calculated using the following equation for a Gaussian-shaped peak:

$N = 16(tr/W)^2$

where:

- tr = retention time
- W = peak width at base

van Deemter equation

The van Deemter equation relates the theoretical plate height, or efficiency, of a chromatographic column to the various flow and kinetic parameters which cause peak broadening, as follows:

$HETP = A + B/u + C \cdot u$

where:

- HETP = height equivalent to a theoretical plate, a measure of the dispersion value of the column [m]
- A = Eddy-diffusion parameter, related to channeling through a non-ideal packing [m]
- B = diffusion coefficient of the eluting particles in the longitudinal direction, resulting in dispersion, expressed in $m^2\ s^{-1}$
- C = Resistance to mass transfer coefficient of the analyte between mobile and stationary phase, expressed in seconds (s)
- u = Linear velocity expressed in $m\ s^{-1}$

Index

2D chromatography, 8
3-(4-Hydroxyphenyl)propionic

acid (HPPA), 8
abbreviated new drug application (ANDA), 8
absolute bioavailability, 8
absorption, 9
absorption, distribution, metabolism and excretion (ADME), 9
accelerator mass spectrometry, 9
acceptance criteria, 9
accuracy, 10
accurate mass, 10
acid dissociation, 10
adverse event, 10
affinity, 11
affinity-based biosensor, 11
AI performance monitoring, 11
alignment, 12
ambient ionization, 12
analyte, 12
analyte fortification, 12
analytical procedure, 13
analytical range, 13
analytical run, 13
anchor calibrator, 13
antibody, 14
antibody-drug conjugate (ADC), 14
anticoagulant, 14
antidrug antibody (ADA), 14
antigen, 14
anti-idiotypic antibody, 15
antisense oligonucleotide, 15
aptamer, 15
aqueous normal-phase liquid chromatography (ANP-LC), 15
archive, 16
area under the curve (AUC), 16
artificial intelligence (AI), 17
assay, 17
assay development, 17
assay-appropriate scientific validation, 17
atmospheric pressure chemical ionization (APCI), 18
audit, 18
audit trail, 18
automation, 19
autosampler, 19
autosampler stability, 19

back-calculation, 19
balance, 19
basal value, 20
baseline, 20
batch, 20
bench-top stability, 20
between run, 20

bias, 21
bioanalysis, 21
bioassay, 21
bioavailability, 21
biobetter, 23
biocompatibility, 23
biodistribution, 23
bioequivalence, 23
bioinert, 24
bioinformatics, 24
biolayer interferometry, 24
biologic/biotherapeutic/biopharmaceutical, 24
biological matrix, 25
biologics license application (BLA), 25
biomanufacturing, 25
biomarker, 25
biosensor, 26
biosimilar, 26
biotransformation, 27
bispecific therapeutic proteins, 27
Bland–Altman plot, 27
blank sample, 27
blood:plasma distribution ratio, 28
blood–brain barrier, 28
bottom-up proteomics, 28
bradford assay, 28
bridging immunoassay, 29

calibration curve, 29
calibration range, 29
calibration standard, 30
candidate surrogate end point, 30
capacity factor, 30
capillary zone electrophoresis, 30
capture capability, 31
carrier protein, 31

carryover, 31
CAR-T cell (or chimeric antigen receptor T cell), 31
cell therapy, 32
cell-based neutralizing antibody assay, 32
Centers for Disease Control and Prevention (CDC), 32
centrifugation, 32
certificate of analysis (CoA), 33
chemiluminescence, 33
chiral chromatography, 33
chiral compound, 33
chiral inversion, 34
chromatogram, 34
chromatographic column, 34
chromatography, 34
clinical benefit, 35
clinical bioanalytical sample, 35
clinical laboratory improvement amendments (CLIA), 35
clinical outcome, 35
clinical trial, 35
clinical utility, 36
clinical validation, 36
co-administered medicines, 36
coefficient of variation (CV), 36
collision-induced dissociation/collision-activated dissociation, 37
comedication stability, 37
companion diagnostic, 37
competitive ligand-binding assay, 38

compliance, 38
computer software validation, 38
conjugation, 38
contamination, 39
context of use (COU) -
biomarkers, 39
contract manufacturing
organization (CMO), 39
contract research organization
(CRO), 39
convergence chromatography, 39
convolutional neural network
(CNN), 40
coronavirus disease (COVID-19), 40
counter ion, 40
CRISPR, 40
critical reagent, 41
cross-reactivity, 41
cross-validation, 41
cumulative urinary excretion curve, 42
curvature, 42
cut point, 42
cytochrome P450, 42

data card, 43
data management, 43
daughter ion, 43
deconvolution, 44
deep learning, 44
derivatization, 45
diagnostic assay, 45
diastereoisomer, 46
difference plot, 46
digestion, 46
digital twin, 46
dilution, 47
dilution QC sample, 47
dilutional linearity , 47
discriminative metabolomics, 47
diversion of LC flow, 48
doping analysis, 48
dosage regimen, 48
dose, 48
dose–response curve, 49
dosing interval, 49
dosing vehicle, 49
dried blood spot (DBS)
sampling, 49
droplet digital PCR (ddPCR), 49
drug metabolism, 50
drug–drug interaction, 50
dry-down, 50

electrochemiluminescence (ECL), 50
electronic workflow, 50
electrospray ionization (ESI), 51
elimination half-life, 51
elution, 51
enantiomer, 51
endogenous compound, 51
endpoint, 52
enzyme, 52
enzyme induction, 52
enzyme inhibition, 52
enzyme-linked immunosorbent
assay (ELISA), 52
epimer, 53
epitope, 53
esterase, 53
European Medicines Agency
(EMA), 53
ex vivo, 53

excretion, 54
extractability, 54
extrapolation, 54

false-negative, 54
false-positive, 55
FDA Form 483, 55
fingerprinting, 55
first-in-human (FIH), 55
first-pass effect, 56
fit-for-purpose, 56
flow cytometry, 56
follow-on biologic, 56
Food and Drug Administration (FDA), 56
formalin-fixed paraffin-embedded (FFPE) tissue specimens, 57
formulation, 57
free drug, 57
free jet expansion, 57
freeze-thaw stability, 58
full validation, 58
functional neutralizing antibody assay, 58

gas chromatography (GC), 58
gene editing, 59
gene therapy, 59
generative AI, 59
generic drug, 59
good clinical practice (GCP), 60
good laboratory practice (GLP), 60
good manufacturing practice (GMP), 60
gradient elution, 60

heartcutting, 61
hematocrit, 61
hemolysis, 61
hepatic clearance, 61
heteroscedasticity, 61
high dose-hook phenomenon, 62
high ionic strength dissociation assay (HISDA), 62
high-performance (or pressure) liquid chromatography (HPLC), 62
high-resolution mass spectrometry (HRMS), 63
high-throughput screening, 63
hit, 63
hit confirmation, 63
hit identification, 64
hit-to-lead/lead generation, 64
homogenate, 64
homogenization, 64
homoscedasticity , 64
Hook effect, 65
hydrophilic interaction liquid chromatography (HILIC), 65
hydrophilic-phase extraction (HPE), 65
hydrophobic interaction liquid chromatography (HIC), 66
hyperlipidemia (lipemia), 66

IC_{50}, 66
ICH M10 (bioanalytical method validation and study sample analysis), 67
immobilization capacity, 67
immunity, 68
immunoaffinity chromatography, 68

immunoaffinity-LC–MS/MS (IA-MS), 68
immunoassay, 69
immunocapture, 69
immunocompromised, 69
immunocytochemistry, 69
immunogen, 70
immunogenicity, 70
immunogenicity assay, 70
immunohistochemistry (IHC), 70
imprecision, 71
in silico, 71
in situ, 71
in vitro, 72
in vivo, 72
inaccuracy, 72
incubation, 72
incurred sample, 72
incurred sample reanalysis, 74
in-source fragmentation, 74
instrument qualification (IQ/OQ/PQ), 75
inter-assay accuracy, 75
inter-assay precision, 76
interference, 76
interim data, 76
intermediate precision, 76
internal standard, 76
International Council for Harmonisation of Technical Requirements for Pharmaceuticals for Human Use (ICH), 77
interpolation, 77
intra-assay accuracy, 77
intra-assay precision, 77
intravascular administration, 78
intrinsic clearance, 78
investigational New Drug (IND) application, 78
investigator's brochure (IB), 78
ion source, 79
ion suppression, 79
ion trap mass spectrometer, 79
ion-exchange chromatography, 79
ion-mobility spectrometry, 79
ion-pairing chromatography, 80
ion-pairing reagent, 80
isobaric isomers, 80
isocratic elution, 81
isotope dilution, 81
isotopologue, 81

kinetics, 81
kosmotropes, 82

lab-on-a-chip, 82
laboratory information management system (LIMS), 82
large language model (LLM), 82
lead candidate, 83
lead optimization, 83
least squares, 83
ligand-binding assay (LBA), 83
limit of detection (LOD), 84
linear regression, 84
lipidomics, 84
liposomal drug, 84
liquid chromatography (LC), 85
liquid–liquid extraction, 85
locked nucleic acid (LNA), 85
long-term stability, 85

lower limit of quantification (LLOQ), 86
luciferase, 86
luciferin, 86
luminometer (or luminescence microplate reader), 86

machine learning, 87
mass accuracy, 87
mass resolution, 87
mass spectrometry, 87
mass-to-charge (m/z), 88
master schedule, 88
matching matrix, 88
matrix, 89
matrix effect, 89
matrix factor (MF), 89
matrix-assisted laser desorption ionization (MALDI), 89
maximum tolerated dose (MTD), 90
mechanism of action (MOA), 90
Medicines and Healthcare products Regulatory Agency (MHRA), 90
metabolite, 91
metabolite features, 91
metabolite profiling, 91
metabolites in safety testing (MIST), 91
metabolome coverage, 92
metabolomic biomarker, 92
metabolomics, 92
meta-metabolomics, 93
method, 93
method development, 93
method qualification, 93
method transfer, 93
method validation, 94
micellar electrokinetic chromatography, 94
micelle, 94
microbore column, 95
micro-elution, 95
microflow, 95
microfluidics, 96
microsample, 96
microsampling, 96
miniature mass spectrometer, 96
minimal residual disease (MRD), 96
minimum required dilution, 97
mixed-mode, 97
mobile phase, 97
molecular ion, 97
molecularly imprinted polymer (MIP), 98
monitoring peptide, 98
monoclonal, 98
monoclonal antibody, 98
monolith, 99
mRNA vaccines, 99
multi ascending dose (MAD), 99
multi-analyte, 100
multiple heartcutting 2D separation, 100
multiple reaction monitoring (MRM), 101
multiplexing, 101
multiply-charge ion, 101
multi-site study, 101

nanoflow, 102
nanoflow liquid chromatography, 102
nanoscience, 102

neutralizing antibody (NAb), 102
New Drug Application (NDA), 103
nominal concentration, 103
non-cell-based neutralizing antibody (NAb) assay, 103
nonspecific adsorption/binding, 104
nontargeted analysis, 104
non-zero calibrator, 104
normal-phase chromatography, 105
novel isoelectric target depletion (ITaD), 105
nuclear magnetic resonance (NMR) spectroscopy, 105

oligonucleotide, 105
online extraction, 106
optimization, 106
oral administration, 106
Organisation for Economic Co-operation and Development (OECD), 106
origin-adjusted approach, 107
orthogonal, 107
out of specification (OOS) investigation, 107
outlier, 108
over-curve concentration, 108
oxidation, 108

pandemic, 108
parallel reaction monitoring (PRM), 109
parallelism, 109
parallel-line analysis (PLA), 109
paratope, 110
parent ion, 110
partial least-squares regression (PLS), 110
partial validation, 111
passivation, 111
patient stratification, 111
peak area, 111
peak area ratio, 112
peak capacity, 112
peak fronting, 112
peak height, 112
peak height ratio, 113
peak tailing, 113
peak tailing factor, 113
PEGylated lipid nanoparticle, 114
per aqueous liquid chromatography, 114
percent difference from theoretical, 114
peripheral blood monouclear cell (PBMC), 114
peripheral compartment, 115
personalized medicine, 115
pharmacodynamics (PD), 115
pharmacogenomics, 115
pharmacokinetics (PK), 116
pharmacology, 116
pharmacometabonomics/ pharmacometabolomics, 116
phase I drug metabolism, 116
Phase I trial, 117
phase II drug metabolism, 117
Phase II trial, 117
Phase III trial, 117
Phase IV trial, 118
phosphatase, 118
phosphodiester, 118

phospholipids, 118
phosphorothioate, 119
phosphorylation, 119
pipette, 119
pKa, 119
placebo, 120
plasma, 120
plasma protein binding, 120
plate reader, 120
point-of-care testing, 121
polyclonal antibodies, 121
polyethylene glycol (PEG), 121
polymerase chain reaction (PCR), 122
population-specific cut point, 122
positive control, 122
post-column infusion, 123
post-market surveillance, 123
post-translational modification (PTM), 123
precipitation and acid dissociation (PandA), 124
precision, 124
precision medicine, 125
preclinical study, 125
precursor ion, 126
predictive metabolomics, 126
pre-digestion liquid chromatography-mass spectrometry with immuno capture (PrD-LC-MS IC), 127
pre-digestion liquid chromatography-mass spectrometry with immuno capture and selective capture (PrD-LC-MS IC SC), 127
pre-digestion liquid chromatography-mass spectrometry with selective capture (PrD-LC-MS SC), 128
pre-dose sample, 128
preventative maintenance (PM), 128
principal components analysis (PCA), 129
principal investigator (PI), 129
processed sample, 129
processing batch, 130
prodrug, 130
product ion, 130
protease, 130
protein binding, 131
protein precipitation, 131
protein quantification, 131
protein therapeutics, 132
proteolysis, 132
proteolytic digestion liquid chromatography-mass spectrometry (PrD-LC-MS), 132
proteomics, 133
protocol, 133
protocol amendment, 133
protocol deviation, 134
proxy matrix, 134
prozone effect, 134

qualified assay, 134
quality assurance, 135
quality control, 135
quality control (QC) sample, 135
quantification range, 135

radioimmunoassay (RIA), 136
raw data, 136
reactive metabolite, 137
reagent, 137
reanalysis, 137

receptor occupancy (RO), 137
recovery (extraction), 138
reference standard, 138
regulated bioanalysis, 138
regulatory validation, 138
reintegration, 138
relative bioavailability, 139
relative error, 139
relative standard deviation (RSD), 139
repeatability, 139
reproducibility, 139
resolution, 140
response function, 140
retention time (RT), 140
reversed-phase chromatography, 140
ribonucleic acid (RNA), 141
risk-based approach, 141
robustness, 141
r-squared, 141
ruggedness, 142

salting out assisted liquid–liquid extraction (SALLE), 142
sample, 142
sample analysis, 142
sample diluent, 143
sample pretreatment, 143
scientific validation, 143
selected reaction monitoring (SRM), 143
selectivity, 144
sensitivity, 144
serum, 144
shotgun proteomics, 144
side effect, 145
signal-to-noise ratio (S/N), 145
significant human metabolite, 145
Simoa® bead technology, 145
single-dose administration, 145
size-exclusion chromatography, 146
solid-phase analytical derivatization, 146
solid-phase extraction (SPE), 146
solubility, 146
specificity, 146
specimen, 147
Spike (noun), 147
spike (verb), 147
spike recovery, 147
stability, 147
stable-labeled isotope, 148
stable-labeled protein, 148
stage-appropriate scientific validation, 148
standard curve, 149
standard operating procedure (SOP), 149
stationary phase, 149
steady state, 149
stock solution, 150
study director, 150
study monitor, 150
study plan, 150
study sample, 151
supercritical fluid chromatography (SFC), 151
superficially porous (core-shell) particle technology, 151
supernatant, 151
supported-liquid extraction, 151

surface plasmon resonance (SPR), 152
surrogate analyte, 152
surrogate matrix, 152
surrogate peptide, 152
surrogate standards, 153
symmetry factor, 153
system priming, 153
system suitability, 153

tandem mass spectrometry, 154
tandem quadrupole mass spectrometry, 154
target, 154
target candidate, 154
target engagement (TE), 155
target validation, 155
targeted analysis, 155
targeted proteomics, 155
targeted quantitation, 156
therapeutic drug monitoring, 156
tiered approach, 156
time-of-flight mass spectrometry (TOF-MS), 156
tissue distribution, 157
top-down proteomics, 157
total drug, 157
total error, 157
total ion chromatogram (TIC), 157
toxicity, 158
transcription, 158
translational research, 158
turbulent flow, 158

ultra-high-performance liquid chromatography (UHPLC), 158
undersampling, 159
unknown, 159
upper limit of quantification (ULOQ), 159

vaccine, 160
validation, 160
validation report, 160
vector, 161
very-high-pressure liquid chromatography (VHPLC), 161
virus, 161
volumetric absorptive microsampling, 161

weighting factor, 161
white paper, 162
whole blood, 162
within-run, 162
World Health Organization (WHO), 162

zero cailibrator, 162

Company profiles

Alturas Analytics
Bioanalytical Experts

Contact details:
1324 Alturas Drive
Moscow
ID 83843
USA
Tel.: +1 208 883 3400
https://alturasanalytics.com

Alturas Analytics is a GLP-compliant bioanalytical contract research organization specializing in LC-MS/MS solutions supporting preclinical and clinical drug development, IND submissions and New Drug Applications. Our business is built on developing long-term collaborations with our clients through a focused emphasis on teamwork, communication and exceptional science.

Alturas has a proven record with complex analyses supporting drug candidates for the pharmaceutical and biotechnology industries. The company operates in a GLP environment using validated operational processes in strict adherence to internal SOPs and applicable global regulations. Our bioanalytical services include:

- Method development and validation
- LC-MS/MS, GC-MS/MS, and HRMS/MS bioanalysis
- Regulated and non-regulated sample analysis in any matrix
- Small molecule, peptide, drug conjugate (e.g., ADCs), and protein based therapeutic (biologics) analysis
- Quantitative biomarker analysis
- Plasma protein binding determinations
- Microsample analysis techniques
- Pharmacokinetic/toxicokinetic analysis and reporting (non-compartmental analysis)
- SEND compliant datasets

Clients have direct access to a team of professionals who understand the critical nature of each project. Our highly skilled scientific team includes innovators of dried blood and matrix spot technology and microflow-LC-MS/MS as routine quantitative techniques supporting regulated studies. At Alturas, we maintain an intensive research effort applying new technologies that lead to scientific advancement and enhanced efficiencies.

KCAS bio
SCIENCE ACCELERATED

Contact details:
10830 S Clay Blair Boulevard
Olathe
KS 66061
USA
Tel.: +1 913 248 3000
https://kcasbio.com

KCAS Bio is a leading bioanalytical contract research organization (CRO) with a proven record of advancing drug development worldwide. We have supported more than 315 FDA-approved drugs, developed over 6,200 proprietary and non-proprietary assays, and successfully completed more than 20 FDA audits with no major findings.

As a top bioanalytical CRO lab, we continually invest in the latest instrumentation and combine this technical expertise with a consultative approach, ensuring our clients' goals are achieved with confidence. Our teams also bring specialized expertise in advanced modalities, allowing us to support the evolving needs of modern drug development. By consistently benchmarking and optimizing our operations, we help scientific innovators and investors move forward with greater certainty.

With facilities across the US and Europe, along with a strategic alliance in Australia, we provide global sponsors with comprehensive services including bioanalytical, biomarker, immunogenicity, cellular and molecular assay capabilities, as well as clinical kitting and sample management.

Bioanalysis author guidelines

About the journal

Bioanalysis is an international, peer-reviewed journal publishing high-quality, review articles, original research, editorials and drug evaluation articles on vaccines. Please see the journal's Aims & Scope for information about its focus and peer-review policy.

These instructions will ensure we have everything required so your paper can move through peer review, production and publication smoothly. Please take the time to read and follow them as closely as possible, as doing so will ensure your paper matches the journal's requirements.

We offer a range of editing, manuscript preparation and post publication services to assist you in preparing your manuscript for submission, increase your chance of acceptance, or broaden the readership of your article. General guidance on every stage of the publication process is available at our Author Services website.

ScholarOne Manuscripts

This journal uses ScholarOne Manuscripts (previously Manuscript Central) to peer review manuscript submissions. Please read the guide for ScholarOne authors before making a submission. Complete guidelines for preparing and submitting your manuscript to this journal are provided below.

Submitting your paper

This journal uses ScholarOne Manuscripts to manage the peer-review process. If you haven't submitted a paper to this journal before, you will need to create an account in the submission centre. Please read these guidelines and then submit your paper in the relevant Author Centre, where you will find user guides and a helpdesk.

This journal accepts article proposals and presubmission enquiries via direct email to the editorial team. Please read these guidelines and then submit your paper to the Commissioning Editor.

Please note that this journal uses Crossref™ to screen papers for unoriginal material. By submitting your paper to *Bioanalysis* you are agreeing to originality checks during the peer-review and production processes.

On acceptance, we recommend that you keep a copy of your Accepted Manuscript.

Open Access

You have the option to publish open access in this journal via our Open Select publishing program. Publishing open access means that your article will be free to access online immediately on publication, increasing the visibility, readership and impact of your research. Articles published Open Select with Taylor & Francis typically receive 35% more citations* and over 5 times as many downloads** compared to those that are not published Open Select.

Your research funder or your institution may require you to publish your article open access. Visit our Author Services website to find out more about open access policies and how you can comply with these.

You will be asked to pay an article publishing charge (APC) to make your article open access and this cost can often be covered by your institution or funder. Use our APC finder to view the APC for this journal. Please note that only the corresponding author is eligible to request funding from their institution, and it is not possible to change the corresponding author to achieve eligibility after submission. For further information, please see details here.

Please visit our Author Services website if you would like more information about our Open Select Program.

*Citations received up to 7th August 2024 for articles published in 2019-2023. Data obtained on 7th August 2024, from Digital Science's Dimensions platform, available at https://app.dimensions.ai
**Usage in 2021-2023 for articles published in 2019-2023.

Article Publishing Charge for Plain Language Summary of Publication (PLSP) and Podcasts

All PLSP in this journal are published on an open access basis so they are freely accessible to all wanting to understand the latest research. Therefore, there is an article publishing charge (APC) to cover the costs associated with publishing the PLSP. The APC to publish a PLSP in this journal is $5,500 / £4,400 / €5,330 / AUD 7,678, plus VAT or other local taxes where applicable in your country. There is no submission charge.

The PLSP APC in this journal covers the following:

- Publishing the PLSP open access under a CC BY-NC-ND license
- Editorial review of the PLSP prior to publication, including internal review, external peer review by patient/lay/plain language experts and editorial feedback (in terms of content, readability and design)
- In-house processing of the PLSP from submission to publication
- Full design of the final article, including creation of additional imagery, re-styling of graphics and layout into a patient-friendly format

- Online hosting of the PLSP with keywords and other tools to enhance discoverability on our journal website and associated Plain Language Summaries website
- Dissemination across social media (X, LinkedIn and Facebook) using relevant hashtags and mentions
- Indexing on relevant database, such as Medline, where applicable (in accordance with the journal's indexing status)
- Liaison with relevant patient organization to ensure they are aware of the PLSP as a tool to educate and inform their members

All Podcasts in this journal are published on an open access basis so they are freely accessible to all wanting to understand the latest research. Therefore, there is an article publishing charge (APC) to cover the costs associated with publishing the podcast article. The APC to publish a Podcast in this journal is $2,500 / £2,000 / €2,423 / AUD 3,490, plus VAT or other local taxes where applicable in your country. There is no submission charge. The podcast article APC in this journal covers the following:

- Publishing the podcast article open access under a CC BY-NC-ND license
- Dissemination across social media (X, LinkedIn and Facebook) using relevant hashtags and mentions
- Indexing on relevant database, such as Medline, where applicable (in accordance with the journal's indexing status)
- Double anonymized peer review of the discussion points, with editorial review of the accepted recording
- Recorded podcast with full transcript to be provided on acceptance of discussion points
- Online hosting of podcast article with keywords and other tools to enhance discoverability on our journal website

Peer review & revision

Taylor & Francis is committed to peer-review integrity and upholding the highest standards of review. Once your paper has been assessed for suitability by the editor, it will then be anonymously peer-reviewed by independent, anonymous expert referees, each delivering at least one report. If you have shared an earlier version of your Author's Original Manuscript on a preprint server or registered your study with a registry (e.g. ClinicalTrials.gov), please be aware that anonymity cannot be guaranteed. Further information on our preprints policy and citation requirements can be found on our Preprints Author Services page. Find out more about what to expect during peer review and read our guidance on publishing ethics.

The following summary describes the peer review process for this journal:

- Identity transparency: double anonymized
- Reviewer interacts with: Editor
- Review information published: none

Preparing your paper

All authors submitting to medicine, biomedicine, health sciences, allied and public health journals should conform to the Uniform Requirements for Manuscripts Submitted to Biomedical Journals, prepared by the International Committee of Medical Journal Editors (ICMJE).

Guidelines by article type

Please follow the Expert Medicine Author Guidelines to view the article types published in this journal and detailed guidelines for each article type.

Formatting

Papers should be submitted in Word format.

File formatting: Keep all formatting to a minimum. Do not assign 'styles' to headings, extracts or paragraphs. Make sure that the 'normal' style is used throughout the text. Turn off the automatic hyphenation feature.

Spacing and headings: Headings, sub-headings and title paragraphs should be used to divide the text. Please use numbers (Arabic numerals) to indicate a hierarchy of headings/sub-headings (i.e., 1.0, 1.1, 2.0, 2.1, 2.1.1, 2.1.2 and so on).

Spelling: All articles will be published in American English. Authors are advised to check their work for English spelling and grammar prior to submission. The Editorial Office can assist with the process of preparing and submitting a manuscript with Taylor & Francis Editing Services, offering authors: English language editing, translation (from Chinese, Spanish, Portuguese or Japanese into English), manuscript formatting and figure preparation.

Please see our formatting guide for full instructions.

References

Please use this reference guide when preparing your paper. An EndNote output style is also available to assist you.

Papers or patents of particular interest should be identified using one or two asterisk symbols (* = of interest, ** = of considerable interest), and annotated with a brief sentence explaining why the reference is considered to be of interest.

Using third-party material in your paper

You must obtain the necessary permission to reuse third-party material in your article. The use of short extracts of text and some other types of material is usually permitted, on a limited basis, for the purposes of criticism and review without securing formal permission. If you wish to include any material in your paper for which you do not hold copyright, and which is not covered by this informal agreement, you will need to obtain written permission from the copyright owner prior to submission. More information on requesting permission to reproduce work(s) under copyright.

Financial and competing interests disclosure

Please include a disclosure of interest statement, using the subheading "Financial and competing interests disclosure." If you have no interests to declare, please state this (suggested wording: The authors report no conflicts of interest). For all NIH/Wellcome-funded papers, the grant number(s) must be included in the disclosure of interest statement. Read more on disclosing conflicts of interest.

Clinical Trials Registry

In order to be published in a Taylor & Francis journal, all clinical trials must have been registered in a public repository, ideally at the beginning of the research process (prior to participant recruitment). Trial registration numbers should be included in the abstract, with full details in the methods section. Clinical trials should be registered prospectively – i.e. before participant recruitment. However, for clinical trials that have not been registered prospectively, Taylor & Francis journals requires retrospective registration to ensure the transparent and complete dissemination of all clinical trial results which ultimately impact human health. Authors of retrospectively registered trials must be prepared to provide further information to the journal editorial office if requested. The clinical trial registry should be publicly accessible (at no charge), open to all prospective registrants, and managed by a not-for-profit organization. For a list of registries that meet these requirements, please visit the WHO International Clinical Trials Registry Platform (ICTRP). The registration of all clinical trials facilitates the sharing of information among clinicians, researchers, and patients, enhances public confidence in research, and is in accordance with the ICMJE guidelines.

Complying with ethics of experimentation

Please ensure that all research reported in submitted papers has been conducted in an ethical and responsible manner, and is in full compliance with all relevant codes of experimentation and legislation. All original research papers involving humans, animals, plants, biological material, protected or non-public datasets, collections or sites, must include a written statement in the Methods section, confirming ethical approval has been obtained from the appropriate local ethics committee or Institutional Review Board and that where relevant, informed consent has been obtained. For animal studies, approval must have been obtained from the local or institutional animal use and care committee. All research studies on humans (individuals, samples, or data) must have been performed in accordance with the principles stated in the Declaration of Helsinki. In settings where ethics approval for non-interventional studies (e.g. surveys) is not required, authors must include a statement to explain this. In settings where there are no ethics committees in place to provide ethical approval, authors are advised to contact the Editor to discuss further. Detailed guidance on ethics considerations and mandatory declarations can be found in our Editorial Policies section on Research Ethics.

Consent

All authors are required to follow the ICMJE requirements and Taylor & Francis Editorial Policies on privacy and informed consent from patients and study participants. Authors must include a statement to confirm that any patient, service user, or participant (or that person's parent or legal guardian) in any type of qualitative or quantitative research, has given informed consent to participate in the research. For submissions where patients or participants can be potentially identified (e.g. a clinical case report detailing their medical history, identifiable images or media content, etc), authors must include a statement to confirm that they have obtained written informed consent to publish the details from the affected individual (or their parents/guardians if the participant in not an adult or unable to give informed consent; or next of kin if the participant is deceased). The process of obtaining consent to publish should include sharing the article with the individual (or whoever is consenting on their behalf), so that they are fully aware of the content of the article before it is published. Authors should familiarise themselves with our policy on participant/patient privacy and informed consent. They may also use the Consent to Publish Form, which can be downloaded from the same Author Services page.

Health and safety

Please confirm that all mandatory laboratory health and safety procedures have been complied with in the course of conducting any experimental work reported in your paper. Please ensure your paper contains all appropriate warnings on any hazards that may be involved in carrying out the experiments or procedures you have described, or that may be involved in instructions, materials, or formulae.

Please include all relevant safety precautions; and cite any accepted standard or code of practice. Authors working in animal science may find it useful to consult the International Association of Veterinary Editors' Consensus Author Guidelines on Animal Ethics and Welfare and Guidelines for the Treatment of Animals in Behavioural Research and Teaching.

Data Sharing Policy

This journal applies the Taylor & Francis Basic Data Sharing Policy. Authors are encouraged to share or make open the data supporting the results or analyses presented in their paper where this does not violate the protection of human subjects or other valid privacy or security concerns.

Authors are encouraged to deposit the dataset(s) in a recognized data repository that can mint a persistent digital identifier, preferably a digital object identifier (DOI) and recognizes a long-term preservation plan. If you are uncertain about where to deposit your data, please see this information regarding repositories.

Authors are further encouraged to cite any data sets referenced in the article and provide a Data Availability Statement.

At the point of submission, you will be asked if there is a data set associated with the paper. If you reply yes, you will be asked to provide the DOI, pre-registered DOI, hyperlink, or other persistent identifier associated with the data set(s). If you have selected to provide a pre-registered DOI, please be prepared to share the reviewer URL associated with your data deposit, upon request by reviewers.

Where one or multiple data sets are associated with a manuscript, these are not formally peer reviewed as a part of the journal submission process. It is the author's responsibility to ensure the soundness of data. Any errors in the data rest solely with the producers of the data set(s).

Publication charges

For invited content there are no submission fees or page charges.

Colour figures will be reproduced in colour in your online article free of charge.

Please see section Article Publishing Charge for Plain Language Summary of Publications (PLSP) and Podcasts above for details of publication charges which relate to these article types.
When a product has not yet been approved by an appropriate regulatory body for the use described in your paper, please specify this, or that the product is still investigational.

Accelerated Publication

As part of our responsive approach to publishing timely research results, an optional, Accelerated Publication service is available.

- Accelerated Publication: Receive a final decision in as little as 7 weeks* from submission (subject to a 2 week turnaround of the revised paper by the authors, peer review within approximately 4 weeks). Online publication usually occurs 2-3 weeks after acceptance, with first proofs provided within 5 working days. The publication support fee is $3,900/ €3,400/ £3,000 per article.

Acceptance of articles is driven entirely by editorial considerations and independent peer review.

Copyright options

Copyright allows you to protect your original material, and stop others from using your work without your permission. Taylor & Francis offers a number of different license and reuse options, including Creative Commons licenses when publishing open access.

Interviews

Our in-house commissioning editors conduct and write up interviews with key opinions leaders regarding their recent research. These are conducted either via e-mail or on the phone. If you are interested in being interviewed please contact the Commissioning Editor of the journal; their contact details can be found on the journal's homepage.

My Authored Works

On publication, you will be able to view, download and check your article's metrics (downloads, citations and Altmetric data) via My Authored Works on Taylor & Francis Online. This is where you can access every article you have published with us, as well as your free eprints link, so you can quickly and easily share your work with friends and colleagues. We are committed to promoting and increasing the visibility of your article. Here are some tips and ideas on how you can work with us to promote your research.

Queries

Should you have any queries, please visit our Author Services website.

Checklist: what to include

1. **Author details.** Please ensure everyone meeting the International Committee of Medical Journal Editors (ICJME) requirements for authorship is included as an author of your paper. Please ensure all listed authors meet the Taylor & Francis authorship criteria. All authors of a manuscript should include their full name and affiliation on the cover page of the manuscript. Where available, please also include ORCiDs and social media handles (Facebook, X or LinkedIn). One author will need to be identified as the corresponding author, with their email address normally displayed in the article PDF (depending on the journal) and the online article. Authors' affiliations are the affiliations where the research was conducted. If any of the named co-authors moves affiliation during the peer-review process, the new affiliation can be given as a footnote. Please note that no changes to affiliation can be made after your paper is accepted. Read more on authorship.
2. A structured **abstract** of no more than 200 words. A structured abstract should cover (in the following order):
   - Introduction: Authors are required to describe the significance of the topic under discussion.
   - Areas covered: Authors are required to describe the research discussed and the literature search undertaken.
   - Expert Opinion/Commentary: Authors are required to summarise briefly their Expert Opinion/Commentary section. References must not be included in the abstract.Read tips on writing your abstract.
3. **Plain Language Summary.** Taylor & Francis welcomes the submission of plain language summaries (PLS) alongside your manuscript. Please visit the Plain Language Summaries Author Services page to read our PLS Author Guidelines, which discuss developing, submitting, and publishing PLS, and view recent examples of published PLS. Alternatively, Taylor & Francis also welcomes the submission of standalone Plain Language Summary of Publication (PLSP) articles, which are published separately to the original article.
4. You can opt to include a **video abstract** with your article. Find out how these can help your work reach a wider audience, and what to think about when filming. Taylor & Francis Editing Services provides a video abstract creation service for a fee.
5. 5-8 **keywords**. Read making your article more discoverable, including information on choosing a title and search engine optimization.
6. **Funding details.** Please supply all details required by your funding and grant-awarding bodies as follows: *For single agency grants:* This work was supported by the <Funding Agency> under Grant <number xxxx>. *For multiple agency grants:* This work was supported by the <Funding Agency 1> under Grant <number xxxx> <Funding Agency 2> under Grant <number xxxx> and <Funding Agency 3> under Grant <number xxxx>.
7. **Disclosure statement.** This is to acknowledge any financial or non-financial interest that has arisen from the direct applications of your research. If there are no relevant competing interests to declare please state this within the article, for example: The authors report there are no competing interests to declare. Further guidance on what is a conflict of interest and how to disclose it.
8. **Geolocation information.** Submitting a geolocation information section, as a separate paragraph before your acknowledgements, means we can index your paper's study area accurately in JournalMap's geographic literature database and make your article more discoverable to others. More information.
9. **Data availability statement.** If there is a data set associated with the paper, please provide information about where the data supporting the results or analyses presented in the paper can be found. Where applicable, this should include the hyperlink, DOI or other persistent identifier associated with the data set(s). Templates are also available to support authors.
10. **Data deposition.** If you choose to share or make the data underlying the study open, please deposit your data in a recognized data repository prior to or at the time of submission. You will be asked to provide the DOI, pre-reserved DOI, or other persistent identifier for the data set.
11. **Supplemental online material.** Supplemental material can be a video, fileset, audio file or anything which supports (and is pertinent to) your paper. We publish supplemental material online via Figshare. Find out more about supplemental material and how to submit it with your article. Taylor & Francis Editing Services can help you create research promotion materials, including infographics, video abstracts, lay summaries and graphical abstracts, to support your article's impact. For more information, including pricing, visit this website.
12. A maximum of five **figures.** Figures should be high quality (1200 dpi for line art, 600 dpi for grayscale and 300 dpi for colour, at the correct size). Figures should be supplied in one of our preferred file formats: PS, JPEG, TIFF, or Microsoft Word (DOC or DOCX) files are acceptable for figures that have been drawn in Word. For information relating to other file types, please consult our Submission of electronic artwork.
13. A maximum of five **tables**. Tables should present new information rather than duplicating what is in the text. Readers should be able to interpret the table without reference to the text. Please supply editable files.
14. **Equations**. If you are submitting your manuscript as a Word document, please ensure that equations are editable. More information about mathematical symbols and equations.
15. **Units**. Please use SI units (non-italicized).

For all print-only, online-only or print & online subscription queries, please contact Andrea.Fejszes@tandf.co.uk

Indexing: Impact factor: 1.8 (2024), CiteScore: 3.4 (2024), 5 year IF 2.0 (2024). 41 of 79 (Biochemical Research Methods); 37 of 84 (Chemistry, Analytical). Q2 CiteScore Best Quartile. SNIP 0.671 (2024). SJR 0.437 (2024).

BIOSIS Previews; BIOSIS Reviews Reports and Meetings; Chemical Abstracts; EMBASE/Excerpta Medica; Essential Science Indicators; Journal Citation Reports/Science Edition; MEDLINE/Index Medicus; Research Alert; Science Citation Index Expanded (SciSearch®); Scopus.

REPRINTS

Article reprints are available through our reprint service. Please contact Sam.Cavana@tandf.co.uk

CRITICAL REVIEWS IN CLINICAL LABORATORY SCIENCES

VOLUME 62, ISSUE 7 202
ISSN: 0040-50

Impact Factor: 5.5 (2024)
5 year IF: 7.9 (2024)
CiteScore (Scopus): 13.2 (2024)

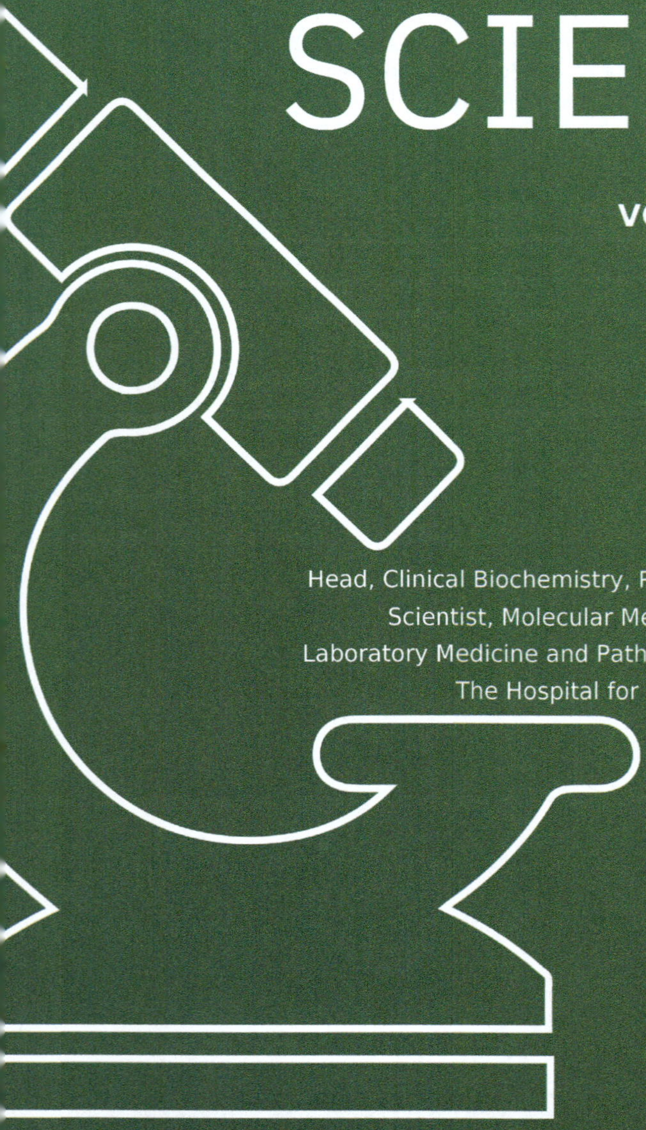

Taylor & Francis
Taylor & Francis Group

9781041162384